M000103999

THIS JOURNAL BELONGS TO:

birth wisdom yoga

remedies and journal

A complete prenatal yoga flow and guide
for beginners to advanced

with Julia Piazza
BA, CD(DONA), E-RYT 200, RPYT

First edition 2017

ISBN 978-0-692-93409-8

SOURCES:
  ACOG-The American College of Obstetricians and Gynecologists

RESOURCES FOR PREGNANCY, BIRTH AND MOTHERING:
  Ecstatic Birth (e-book) Sarah Buckley
  Ina May Gaskin's Guide to Natural Childbirth by Ina May Gaskin
  "Orgasmic Birth" Movie
  Birthing From Within, Pam England & Rob Horowitz
  The Nursing Mother's Companion by Kathleen Huggins
  Healthy Sleep Habits, Happy Child by Marc Weissbluth
  Women's Bodies, Women's Wisdom by Christiane Northrop
  Childbirth Connection
  evidencebasedbirth.com
  lesliehowardyoga.com
  spinningbabies.com

DESIGN:
Lora Watts

PHOTOS:
Michelle MacDonnell Photography

For information about special discounts for bulk purchases, trainings, and/ or appearances at live events, please contact Julia Piazza, julia@birthwisdomyoga.com.

BirthWisdomYoga.com

It is necessary for you to ask your health care provider if it is safe for you and your baby to practice prenatal yoga at this time.

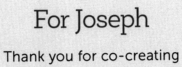

For Joseph

Thank you for co-creating
all things Inspiring with me.

table of contents

acknowledgments

This book was a seed planted by my mother in her constant belief and celebration of women's wisdom, strength and intuition. That seed was later nurtured and bloomed with the birth of each of my children. Thank you, Stetten, Savannah, and Sam for guiding me into my Birth Wisdoms and sharing this Adventure of Life with me. I am deeply humbled by the sacredness of your lives being placed in my hands, and the gift of watching you soar into who you are.

I would like to thank my husband, Joseph, for believing in Birth Wisdom Yoga and for the countless hours of conversation, editing, formatting and support as I gained clarity creating this book.

I am grateful to my collegiate bookends. From Professor Lue Cobene of Solano Community College to Professor Jack Hicks of University of California at Davis, you saw me as a published author long before I shared the same vision.

To the hundreds of Birth Wisdom Prenatal and Postpartum Yoga students, "Dudelas," and Doula Clients: Thank you for inviting me into your lives as you found your voices and pathways to your babies. It has truly been a gift to my life.

My dear sisters Laura, Debbie, Aunt Sally, Giovanna, Shiloh, Gail, Mary, and Michelle, thank you for cheering me on when this book was only an idea and for continuing to encourage me every step of the way. Thank you to Larry, Greg, and my friends and family who have given me endless support and love as I journeyed through life, and believed me when I said this book was "marinating," during years that life events took precedent over writing.

Sisterfriend Natalie, you and Greg inspired me to live my passion in every moment of my life. I am so grateful to know you.

To Lora Watts, Graphic Designer Extraordinaire: Your unlimited talent and vision have captured a lifelong dream of creating Birth Wisdom Yoga and brought it to life on these pages. I am deeply grateful.

To Erica Ramos, I am grateful for your willingness to be a part of this project. The beauty of your spirit and your yoga practice shines through in every photo.

Being a Labor and Delivery Nurse, I thought I was prepared for my own childbirth. Thankfully, I decided to take Birth Wisdom Prenatal Yoga classes in preparation for my delivery, because I could not have gotten through without it. Julia would remind us in class that the only thing you can control in labor is your breath, and that is the TRUTH! I respect Julia's outlook on a "natural delivery." Julia teaches women to trust in the birthing process and to trust in themselves. I wish all of my patients had a copy of *Birth Wisdom Yoga Remedies and Journal,* so that they can walk into the delivery room empowered, educated, and equipped to trust in the birth process, themselves, and their bodies. I can't wait to use this guide with my next pregnancy and gift it to all of my friends! What an amazing tool for mamas!
—*Jennifer Genovese RN, BSN*

Birth Wisdom Yoga Remedies and Journal is a wonderful guide for anyone interested in prenatal yoga and pregnancy. Julia Piazza, a certified labor and birth doula and prenatal yoga instructor, thoughtfully demonstrates specific yoga poses safe for the health of both mother and baby during the different stages of pregnancy. I encourage women at all levels of yoga experience to read this book to learn how the body changes with pregnancy and how yoga can help ease many discomforts that come along with these changes. Reading this book is the next best thing to being in the studio with Julia. —*Fallon Lopez PA-C, MSPAS*

Julia's Birth Wisdom Prenatal Yoga classes have been such a precious gift during my pregnancies and the birth of my children. As a nurse practitioner, I have an understanding of labor and delivery and all of the different interventions that can be involved. However, I also know that many times with interventions, come more interventions. I knew I wanted to try for a non-medicated, vaginal birth with my first child. After Julia's prenatal yoga classes, I felt so prepared and present during labor and delivery. I could hear Julia's voice during the contractions reminding me to breathe and soften my jaw. I had a great first labor and delivery and couldn't wait to do it again. My second pregnancy was a different experience since I was carrying twins. I remember Julia telling me "natural birth is what comes naturally to you" when I told her I would probably be having an epidural due to possible breech extraction. Julia reminded me that "there is pain with a purpose in labor and childbirth, and then there is pain that is suffering." Julia's classes empowered me to "own my birth experience," and although there were multiple interventions that day, I felt present and safe. Everything that makes Julia's prenatal yoga classes so special is right here in *Birth Wisdom Yoga Remedies and Journal.* Now women everywhere can experience the power of Birth Wisdom Yoga in labor, childbirth and mothering. —*Emily Lash, FNP-BC*

midwife foreword

I am thrilled to see Julia's words of wisdom in this gift of a book for childbearing families. She has drawn on ancient traditions and her personal and professional experiences to create a rich guide for health and life. The book prompts women to nourish themselves, and therefore their families, with simple but effective activities including writing prompts and yoga poses organized by trimester.

Self-care is too often low or last on a parent's to-do list, which prioritizes children and leaves little time for much else after work in and outside the home. This book is an antidote with suggestions for quick and powerful ways to focus on presence, breath, movement, and emotional expression to connect with your self and baby while scrap-booking pregnancy mementos, preparing for a healthy birth, and practicing skills that will support parenting in relationship and community.

If there is one thing I've learned as a midwife and mother, it's that families are stronger when parents' love for their children motivates healthy habits and robust self-care practices. The tools that Julia has provided in this gem of a book are not only time tested but research evidence-based. Suggested activities range from exercise with demonstrable physical and psychological benefits, to mindfulness practices which promote wellness and cultivate empathy.

I am grateful to Julia for creating this beautiful guide to well-being, and thank her readers for taking this step to support themselves through the most challenging and wonderful journey of parenthood — Our communities and future will be healthier as a result!

Appreciatively,

Jenna Shaw-Battista
PhD, RN, NP, CNM, FACNM

OB foreword

I was delighted when asked to introduce this lovely book. Julia and I have come to know one another through our shared passion — helping and working with women through the exciting and transformative time of pregnancy and childbirth.

The experience and practice of wellness can mean different things, and I have found that many women struggle with the changes brought by motherhood. Pregnancy is a unique time when the body speaks very loudly — this can be inspiring, scary, confusing, and wonderful all at once. Yoga is a wonderful tool to manage, relieve, or even prevent common pregnancy concerns such as back and leg pain, pelvic discomfort, and anxiety. In addition, both scientific studies and common sense suggest that women who stay active during pregnancy and are mentally, emotionally and physically prepared often have a safer, more effective labor with fewer interventions. Every labor is unique and the more a woman can tap into her individual strength and resilience, the more likely she is to have a positive birth experience for herself and her baby.

I feel very lucky to have Birth Wisdom Yoga as a trusted resource to which I can refer my patients. I love hearing stories from them about how Julia's yoga classes have helped them both physically and emotionally. They are often equally as grateful to have found such lasting connections with other women in their community. I am glad to know that women all over the world will now get to benefit from Julia's wisdom through this thoughtful and thorough guide. Filled with clear photos and detailed recommendations for modifications, this book will serve every woman from those new to yoga looking for a safe way to exercise in pregnancy, to the experienced yogi wondering how to keep her practice going. Enjoy, and I wish you a safe and healthy journey to motherhood!

Hailey R. MacNear, MD
Obstetrician-Gynecologist
Folsom, California

introduction

As I was journeying through my own pregnancies, I gathered wisdoms and inspirations from various sources, including spiritual masters, contemporary teachers and the collective of women who willingly shared their support with me. As I internalized these gifts from others, I became hungry to know more about myself as an individual and about my eventual birth experiences.

Birth Wisdom Yoga Remedies and Journal was created from an inspiration to gift to other women in a single volume the collective wisdom shared with me. It is my soul's gift to you and our "sisters in motherhood," as we journey together through the stages of pregnancy, birth and mothering.

Birth Wisdom Yoga Remedies and Journal will provide you with a map for your pregnancy. In this guided journey, there is a complete prenatal yoga class flow with 35 poses and modifications for the beginning and advanced yoga practitioner. The proper modifications and benefits of each pose are completely explained to keep you and your baby safe, while also preparing you for the "marathon of childbirth." Each trimester of pregnancy and yoga is explained with the common pregnancy ailments and their yoga remedies. The eight Birth Wisdoms are the distinguishing feature of my work: a collection of wisdoms and experiences shared with me over the years as I served women and their families in the labor and birth room, while simultaneously physically and spiritually experiencing the births and growth of my own family.

Also within each Birth Wisdom are meditations and affirmations, along with breathing and softening techniques that will help you find your focal point during labor and childbirth. By adding the poses over the course of your pregnancy as a daily practice, you will be prepared for whatever the path of labor and delivery is for you. The prenatal yoga poses are presented to you in the order that I provide to my students in class. If you are currently a practicing yoga student, the entire flow is listed in the back of the book for you to begin immediately, while using the weekly photos and modifications as needed. If you are a beginning yoga student, work through the poses week to week. As your body feels stronger you will add new poses weekly, working up to the complete flow at the end of the book.

At the end of each week of pregnancy, there are two full journal pages with journal prompts to prepare you mentally for childbirth. Additional space is included for insights, questions, notes to your baby, photos of ultrasound scans and special mementos. You will be creating a keepsake book to save and cherish. I encourage you to use the journaling prompts and space provided to record how you feel. We often find comfort and clarity when we create space for journaling.

A special Labor and Delivery section includes Birth Wisdom Yoga Poses for Labor and Childbirth with special excerpts for the birth partner from my Birth Partner and "Dudela" training workshops. Guidelines for peacefully advocating for mom and baby in the birthing room are included as well.

The book concludes with a comprehensive list of affirmations to take with you to use in labor and childbirth. There is also an additional 30-minute Birth Wisdom Prenatal Yoga flow with balancing and yin yoga poses.

Julia Piazza

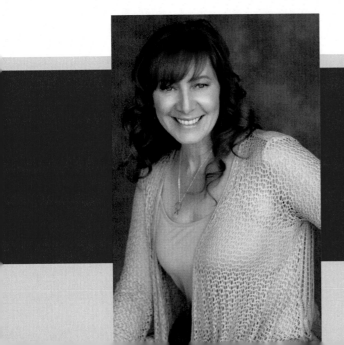

Julia Piazza

Mother of Three Children
B.A., UC Davis
Birth Doula, CD(DONA)
E-RYT 200, RPYT

BirthWisdomYoga.com

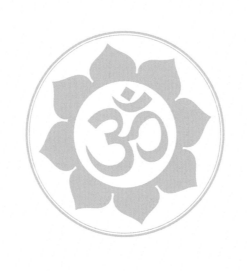
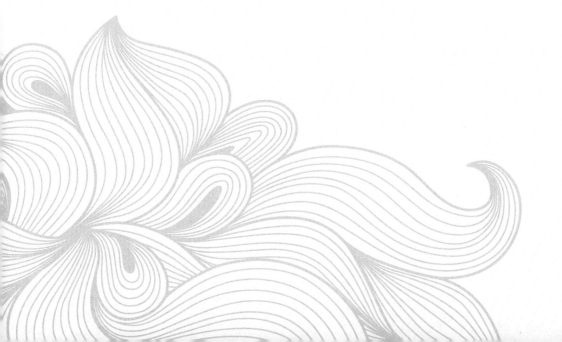

first
trimester
of pregnancy

CONCEPTION TO WEEK 13

Emotionally and spiritually, the first trimester is a time of excitement and wonder. While you may feel ecstatic to be pregnant, it is common to simultaneously feel nervous or anxious about birth and mothering. Fatigue can be a real challenge and is described by many women as feeling like a "blanket of fatigue" that stays with them throughout the day. Physically, as your baby's body structure and organ systems develop, your body is undergoing major changes to support your growing baby. Napping or even just lying down for 30 minutes at a time will be important to support your mind and body during such an exciting time.

You can begin practicing for labor right now, by simply listening to how you feel and creating space for what you need. If you are tired, take a nap or even just lie down and find rest. If you are used to getting things done and pride yourself in efficiency, then prioritizing yourself in this way can be challenging. Meeting this challenge is important practice not only for labor, but also for mothering. Surrendering to what you feel and listening to what you need may include letting things go and *being* rather than *doing*.

FIRST TRIMESTER OF PREGNANCY AND YOGA

- Due to the pregnancy hormone relaxin in the joints, take extra care when stretching, especially in hip-openers.

- Birth Wisdom Yoga Birth Breathing and Ujjayi breathing are safe while practicing yoga. Over time, it is important to practice Birth Wisdom Birth Breathing to prepare for labor and childbirth while simultaneously practicing the yoga poses, since it is the optimal breath to use in labor.

- Drinking plenty of fluids while practicing yoga will help ensure mom is not dehydrated, something that can later stall labor.

- Hot yoga classes are not recommended by most care providers during pregnancy due to the prolonged heat in the yoga room during classes. If you are currently practicing hot yoga, some care providers will ask you to wear a body temperature monitor to make sure your body temperature does not rise above 100°F.

- Breathe, feel, and listen to your body during your yoga practice, remembering if it doesn't feel good, don't do it.

YOGA POSES TO DISCONTINUE DURING THE FIRST TRIMESTER

- Abdominal strengthening poses
- Breath of Fire or forceful breathing
- Poses that require lying on your belly
- Any pose that does not feel good

first trimester common ailments & birth wisdom yoga remedies

POSES FOR SCIATICA AND LOWER BACK PAIN

- Downward Facing Dog
- Pigeon
- Standing 1/2 Moon (with a block, on the wall)
- Bridge and Supported Bridge
- Seated Wide-Legged Straddle
- Narrow Knees Child's Pose (with room for your baby)
- Low Lunges with a blanket under knee on mat. Gently rock forward and back, opening up hips and lower back.

POSES TO AVOID WITH SCIATICA PAIN

- Goddess and Goddess Squat (try chair pose instead for strengthening, with feet hip-width apart)
- Horse
- Wide Leg Child's Pose

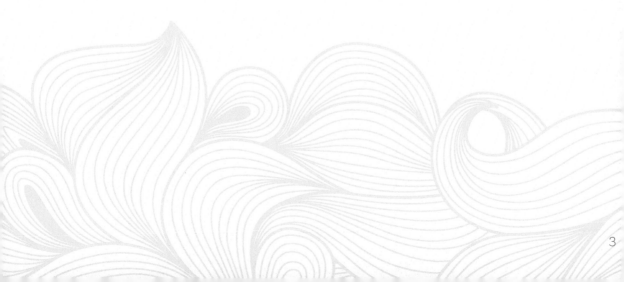

THE PELVIC FLOOR
& PREGNANCY

It is important to know that Kegel exercises are not the best way to strengthen the pelvic floor for pregnancy and childbirth. The latest research on the pelvic floor shows the focus should be on lengthening and strengthening the pelvic floor muscles, rather than squeezing and tightening. Tight pelvic floor muscles can result in an imbalance and weakening of the pelvic floor, resulting in incontinence, pelvic pain and pain with sexual intercourse. For more information on women, the pelvic floor, and yoga, visit www.lesliehowardyoga.com.

There are many Physical Therapists who now specialize in treating women and the pelvic floor. If you experience any pain or discomfort after six weeks postpartum, find a PT in your area.

The optimal exercise for preparing the pelvic floor for labor and delivery begins in Goddess Pose. If your heels do not reach your mat, come into a seated position or lie on your left or right side for comfort and stability.

The pelvic floor and diaphragm flow together when we breathe. When you inhale, the diaphragm and pelvic floor release and drop. When you exhale, the diaphragm and pelvic floor lift. Take a deep inhale – and on your exhale, release the breath completely. With eyes closed, begin to picture the perineum and pelvic floor muscles releasing and softening as you inhale.

As you exhale, gently lift (without squeezing) the pelvic floor muscles up and through the crown of your head. Notice if you are squeezing or tightening, and focus on gentle, slow, lifting instead. Continue to practice the breath with the gentle releasing and lifting of the muscles 3-5 times per week.

breathe

If I had only one gift to give you during your labor, it would be the breath. In our breath, we find our birthing power and strength. We also find our ability to go deep inside. Our breath is the only part of our labor that we can control. It is also our pathway to our baby, no matter what our birth experience looks like. Connecting our breath to movement helps us find our birthing rhythm. It is that rhythm that many women say becomes their "lifeline" for staying on top of the contractions.

When I am connected to my breath in my daily life, I find a rhythm in whatever I am experiencing. The breath gives me the ability to pause and feel, and then communicate from an open heart. I use the breath with stillness in meditation, or even just for short moments in my day. When I am sitting, or waiting in line or at a stop light, I can remember to connect with my breath. This allows me to live from my strength, wisdom and feminine power.

{affirmations}

*My birthing strength and power are found in
my ability to go deep inside and connect with my breath,
surrendering to my birth experience.*

*I pause, breathe and feel,
connecting to my unique mothering wisdom.*

*I create space for stillness and breath during
my daily life and mothering by simply
noticing my inhale and exhale throughout my day.*

Give yourself the gift of stillness and breath in your daily life. This might be as simple as breathing deeply and slowly at each stop light when driving, or maybe sitting quietly for just three minutes alone while connecting to your breath. Allow your inhale to slowly flow up to the sky, and your exhale to gently flow down and out your toes.

BIRTH BREATHING

The breath we practice in Birth Wisdom Yoga classes is the optimal breath to use in labor and childbirth. It is long and slow, helping you connect to your rhythm and focal point in labor.

This is what it looks like:

Beginning with the inhale, allow your breath to slowly reach all the way up through the crown of your head. With your exhale, allow the breath to flow gently down, around your baby and out your toes. Use the breath to feel every part of each yoga pose and to stay in the present moment on your mat.

The more we can stay out of our heads, while diving deep inside of the waves of contractions in our bodies, the easier it is to stay on top of the increasing intensity.

Ujjayi yoga breathing can be practiced if it feels good to you, with a transition to Birth Wisdom Yoga Birth Breathing the last few months of pregnancy to prepare for labor and childbirth.

Pranayama techniques that include the need to hold your breath or take forceful breaths that contract your stomach muscles are not recommended during pregnancy.

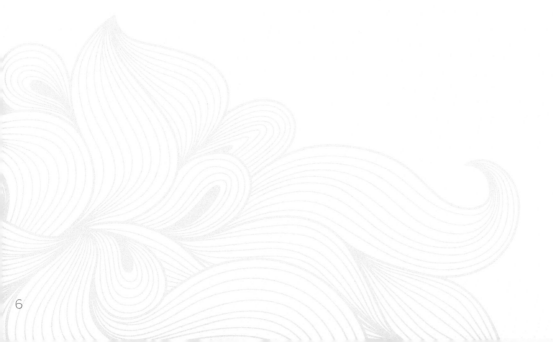

wisdom story
CLEARING SPACE FOR WISDOM

We have many wonderful discussions during sharing circle in our Birth Wisdom Prenatal Yoga classes. The emotions that come up for us during pregnancy, and the gift of space on our yoga mat to release them, are often shared by students. When I think of all the thoughts, plans and worries that we hold onto during pregnancy and mothering, it makes sense that as soon as our forehead meets our mat in child's pose or when we lie in savasana pose, the tears begin to flow. We may resist this feeling of emotion at first, because, we are often taught in our culture that crying should be stopped or avoided by "fixing" the cause of emotion as soon as possible. Well-meaning friends or relatives may try to console us to stop our crying when we show our true feelings.

I have learned that one of the greatest gifts we can give ourselves and our family and friends is permission to cry and express how they feel without "making it better" or offering up solutions. I now think of crying as "clearing space for wisdom." I have found that when I allow myself to pause, breathe and feel what is coming up for me, I am connected to a grounding, authentic energy.

Today, when our 12-year-old son has a difficult day and is crying, I tell him how good it is to release that energy out of his body. This is very different from how I reacted when our two older children would cry at his age. I would try to help them see the positive side of everything, no matter how challenging. Now I just get out of the way and let all three children "feel and clear space for wisdom" before I teach them any lessons in what they are experiencing.

What is one thing you can "get out of the way of" today, allowing yourself to "feel and clear?" This is where you find your strength and your power.

BIRTH WISDOM ONE

reflections, clarifications & mementos

breathe

How can you begin to use the breath in your daily life?

At what part of your day do you find you are holding onto your exhale?

Where can you practice letting go of the breath completely?

What is coming up for you in meditation this week?

Write a letter to your baby.

_____

_____

_____

_____

_____

_____

_____

_____

_____

_____

_____

_____

_____

_____

_____

photos or momentos

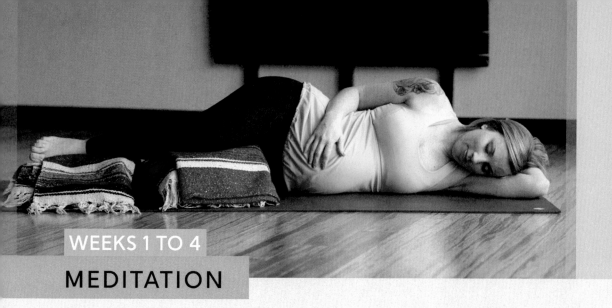

MEDITATION

We begin each Birth Wisdom Yoga class in meditation, lying down on your left or right side, placing a blanket under your head, between your knees or under your baby. Be sure and place a block or blanket between your ankles if you have a blanket between your knees; this will help keep your sciatica nerve from flaring up during pregnancy.

Take a deep inhale. On your exhale, begin to let go of your thoughts, settling into watching the breath completely. Allow your inhale to gently lift up to the sky and your exhale to match the inhale, flowing down, around your baby, and out your toes. Soften your jaw, allow your shoulders to melt away from your ears and sink into your breath even deeper.

Begin to see the beautiful bright light surrounding your entire body – you are discovering your energy field. It's a golden light surrounding you in love and protection, attracting health and abundance to your family. Begin to see that beautiful, golden light flowing to your heart center, and then watch it completely bathe your baby in protective light.

See your baby here, inside of you, in this moment, so content, so peaceful. Everything your baby needs is already right here inside of you. Breathe into the knowing that everything you and your baby need for labor and childbirth is right here inside of you. Soak up this sacred space for you and your baby. Breathe here together, sharing the same breath, sharing the same heartbeat.

After five minutes, take a deep inhale. As you exhale very slowly and gently, find your way onto your hands and knees, placing a blanket in the center of your mat so that when we work on hands and knees, it feels good. Remember to take your time moving through these transitions.

reflections, clarifications &mementos

weeks 1 to 4

photos or momentos

CHILD'S POSE

From Hands and Knees, take your knees as wide as your mat, creating space for your baby. (If your Sciatica Nerve is bothering you, take your knees a little narrower to avoid over-stretching.) Allow your hips to soften down onto your heels. Walk your hands forward, palms down on your mat, and allow your forehead to release all the way down.

Take a deep inhale, and on the exhale let everything go, coming into the breath deeper and slower. This is where you find your birthing strength, in your ability to breathe and feel. If at any time during this practice you feel you have lost the breath, know you can come here or into a seated position to reconnect. — *five breaths* —

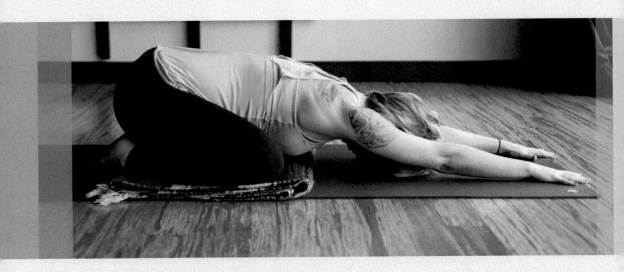

MODIFICATIONS FOR CHILD'S POSE

Place a block under your forehead to bring the earth up to you to soften the stretch. Place a folded blanket or bolster between your sit bones and your heels if there is space.

BENEFITS You have an acupressure point on your forehead that softens and relaxes your entire body in this pose. This is a wonderful place to surrender when you have lost your breath and reconnect before moving on. Yogis call this "Wisdom Pose," because when we lose our breath, our focus, or our stability in another pose, we can rediscover our breath and stability here. It takes wisdom to know when to find rest in all aspects of life.

reflections, clarifications &mementos

week 5

photos or momentos

WEEK 6

LEGS UP THE WALL

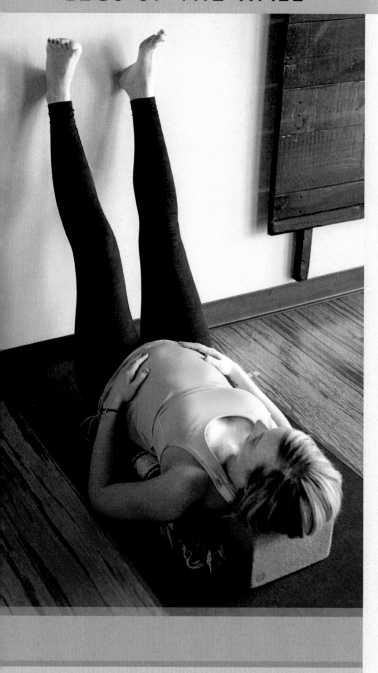

Place two or three blankets under your spine lengthwise, beginning at the sacrum and ending near your shoulders, with a block under your head.

Rest your feet on the wall.
— *five breaths* —

BENEFITS

This pose helps relieve swollen legs and ankles, while promoting healthy circulation. A favorite for many moms after a long day of work.

reflections, clarifications &mementos

week 6

photos or momentos

COW POSE

From hands and knees, knees are hip-width apart, with hands either under your shoulders or slightly forward. Place your blanket in the center of your mat to pad your knees, and with fingers wide for stability, inhale your chin up to the sky, lengthening your spine and exhaling to Cat Pose, arching your back and dropping your head.

MODIFICATIONS Come into a seated position, inhale your chin to the sky, lengthening the spine, and with your exhale round the back softly, tucking your chin. If your wrists feel tight — which is common due to the increase in body fluid during pregnancy — roll up the end of your mat and place your wrist at the fold, taking some weight from the wrist. You can also come onto your fists to lengthen the wrist, if that feels good.

BENEFITS Opens up the lower back, entire spine and neck. Relieves lower back pain, sciatica nerve and hip pain. Creates space for baby and pain relief for mom in any phase of labor and childbirth.

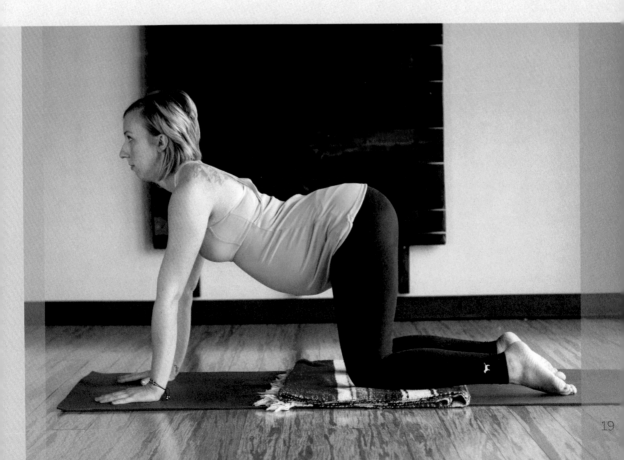

reflections, clarifications &mementos

week 7

photos or momentos

CAT POSE

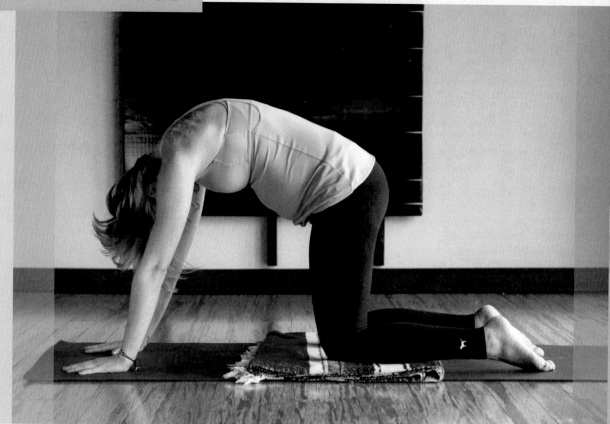

From Cow Pose, with your exhale, press into your hands, arch your back, and tuck your chin. Continue alternating between Cow Pose with your inhale and Cat Pose with your exhale for 3 more sets.

Release to hands and knees.

BENEFITS Opens up the lower back, entire spine and neck. Relieves lower back pain, sciatica nerve and hip pain. Creates space for baby and pain relief for mom in any phase of labor and childbirth.

reflections, clarifications &mementos

week 8

photos or momentos

the simplicity of childbirth

When a woman is guided to listen to what she needs in labor and childbirth, her birth experiences can become an affirmation of lifelong empowerment. The physical support of loving touch and gentle encouragement from her birth partner are key to her finding her way to her baby. Creating a "cocoon-like" environment where lights are dim, voices are low and everyone in the room is supporting mom to find her unique path to her baby gives her the best chance for a natural vaginal labor and childbirth. Allowing mom the space to lead the way and keeping interventions to a minimum should be the focus of her birth partner.

One of the greatest gifts of labor for a mother and her baby is when she discovers that her body and her baby's body are designed to work together in perfect harmony. As your baby sets off signals to tell your body it is the optimal time for labor to begin, contractions make room for your baby to be born as he or she pushes with their feet to move down the birth canal. This unique bond that is created in childbirth will stay in your heart long after labor, reminding you to parent from trust and your body's inner wisdom.

{affirmations}

*My body and my baby's body
work together in perfect harmony.*

*Everything we need for labor, childbirth and mothering
is already right here inside of me.*

RELAXIN AND PRENATAL YOGA

Relaxin is a pregnancy hormone that assists in the softening of the liga-ments, cervix and cartilage in our bodies during pregnancy. It also helps the bones of the pelvis to open during labor.

Relaxin also contributes to the separation of the symphysis pubis, the joint that connects the left and right pubic bones. This separation can cause pain and difficulty in walking, resulting in what is referred to as the "pregnancy waddle." Some women will experience SPD (Symphysis Pubis Dysfunction) in the later months of pregnancy due to the separation of the symphysis pubis joint. Symptoms include a sharp, stabbing pain in the pubic bone area with walking and exercise. See back of book for a quick reference list of yoga remedies for various pregnancy ailments, including SPD.

Relaxin can still be present in your body while you are breastfeeding and even several months afterward, so it is important to take the same precau-tions postpartum as you did prenatally to avoid injury.

YIN POSES TO TAKE SPECIAL CARE WITH DUE TO RELAXIN IN THE JOINTS DURING PREGNANCY

Hip Openers and Yin Poses should not be held for more than 5 breaths at a time to ensure you do not overstretch. Often, if over-stretching or injury has occurred, you may not feel the full severity of it until the following day.

Pigeon : Support your raised hip with a blanket and use a block to "bring the earth up to you and create space for your baby."

Frog on the Wall : Place two or three blankets under your spine lengthwise, beginning at the sacrum and ending near your shoulders, and place a block under your head. Feet are wide on the wall with knees open as wide as feels good in your hips. This creates a wonderful opening for the spine and is safe, because you are not flat on your back or lying on the vena cava artery.

Baddha Konasana : Place blankets under your thighs or knees if needed to support the joints. If your baby is in a Breech position, avoid this pose as it helps create space for baby to engage in the pelvis.

Supta Baddha Konasana : Place two or three blankets under your spine lengthwise, beginning at the sacrum and ending near your shoulders. Place a block under your head. This creates a wonderful opening for the spine and is safe, because you are not lying flat on your back.

Legs up the Wall : This is a great inversion for relieving edema or swelling. Place two or three blankets under your spine lengthwise, beginning at the sacrum and ending towards your shoulders. Place a block under your head.

Rocking Happy Baby Pose : This is a wonderful hip opener and will give you a welcome massage of your spine.

Seated Straddle : Place a blanket under your sit bones, and use a block to rest your forearms or hands on in the center of your mat.

Seated Forward Fold : Legs are as wide as your mat, and your hands rest on your thighs This is a great place for you to use a strap at the ends of your feet and lengthen your spine.

Head to Knee Forward Bend : You can fold forward during your first trimester. In the second and third trimesters, take feet wide and bend the knees deeply while extending the spine forward slowly.

reflections, clarifications &mementos

the simplicity of childbirth

How can you create a "cocoon-like" environment for your labor and birth experience? Make a list of ideas that speak to you. Asking your partner to create a playlist of your favorite songs, planning to use battery operated tea lights to keep the lighting soft, and wearing your own "birthing clothes" may be a place to start.

_____

_____

_____

_____

_____

How will you and your partner prepare to peacefully navigate speaking with hospital staff if interventions are necessary? Review the Informed Consent Questions with your partner (see the Labor Section at the back of the book), and note your thoughts here.

_____

_____

_____

_____

_____

What is coming up for you in meditation this week?

_____

_____

_____

Write a letter to your baby.

_____

_____

_____

_____

_____

_____

_____

_____

_____

_____

_____

_____

photos or momentos

PELVIC CIRCLES

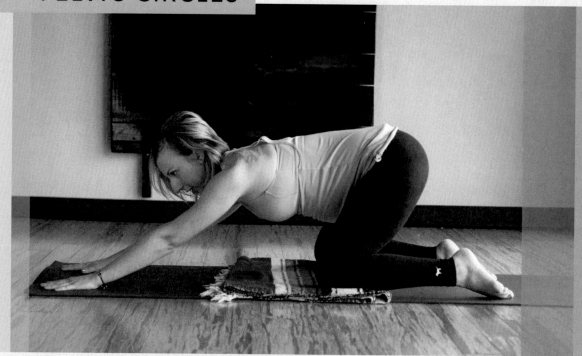

From hands and knees, take your knees almost as wide as your mat and walk your hands forward to create space. Come into pelvic circles to the right and left, making a figure eight with your hips. Take it nice and slow, moving where it feels good in your body. Maybe allow your eyes to close and feel the opening in your hips, lower back and spine.

BENEFITS This entire hands-and-knees sequence helps to ensure your baby is in an optimal position for labor and childbirth by creating space in the pelvis and encouraging your baby into a "head down" position. It is also ideal for any stage of labor, including pushing.

reflections, clarifications &mementos

week 9

photos or momentos

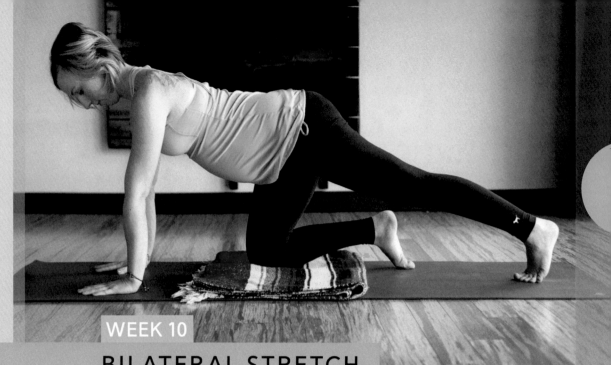

BILATERAL STRETCH

With your hands under your shoulders and your knees under your hips, gently hug your baby into your spine. Place your left foot behind you, press into the ball of your foot, and lengthen your heel toward the back of your mat. Reach your right hand forward, feel the energy from your right fingertips, down your spine and through the heel of your left foot.

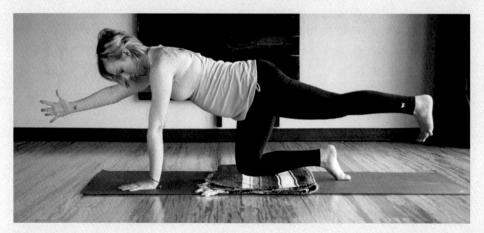

MODIFICATIONS If you are in your first or second trimester and you want to take the pose deeper, slowly lift your left toes off your mat, keeping your left foot in line with your left hip.

BENEFITS Stretches and strengthens the lower back, safely engages and strengthens the core.

reflections, clarifications &mementos

week 10

photos or momentos

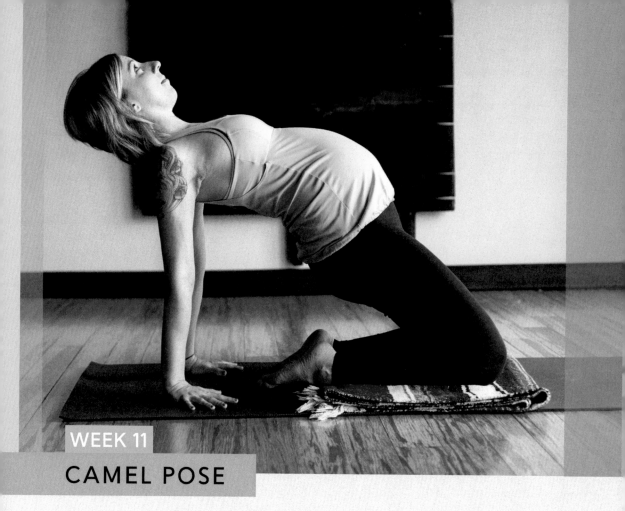

CAMEL POSE

From hands and knees sitting into Hero's Pose with your sit bones resting on your heels, place your hands on your mat behind you with your fingertips facing your toes. Press into your hands, opening your heart and dropping your head back between your shoulder blades or tucking your chin, whichever feels good to you. — *five breaths* —

MODIFICATIONS FOR CAMEL POSE
Sit in an easy seated position if it feels better on your knees with hips down, opening your heart. For a lighter stretch, leave your sit bones on your heels and open the chest.

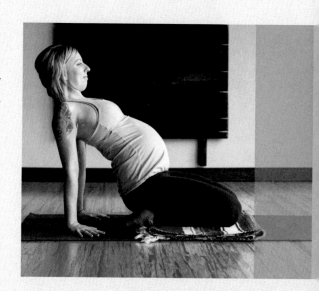

BENEFITS Opens up and stretches the chest, shoulders, neck and spine.

reflections, clarifications &mementos

week 11

photos or moments

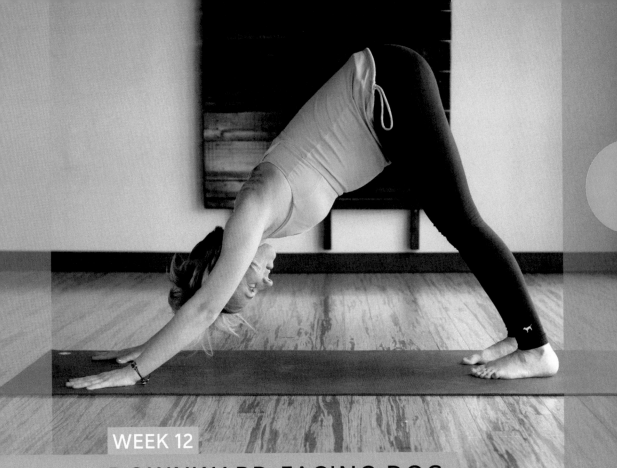

DOWNWARD FACING DOG

From hands and knees, come into Cat Pose, tuck your toes, and press into your hands with fingers wide, lifting your hips to the sky. Hands are shoulder width apart. Take your feet hip width apart, pedal the feet from left to right, and gently move your head yes and no releasing your neck. As you push into your hands feel the length in your spine while your hips reach up to the sky and your heels soften down towards your mat. Three breaths. Take a deep inhale, bend your knees a lot, and walk your hands slowly to your feet standing up.

MODIFICATIONS If Downward Facing Dog feels like too much, use Wall Plank to stretch out your spine. Place your hands at shoulder height and press into the wall. Take your feet wide, step back, and move where it feels good. Maybe bend the right knee, then the left, and find your way into pelvic circles, adjusting the hands higher while using the wall for support.

BENEFITS Lengthens the entire spine, neck and legs. Can be used to help turn a Breech Baby in the last few weeks of pregnancy.

reflections, clarifications &mementos

week 12

photos or momentos

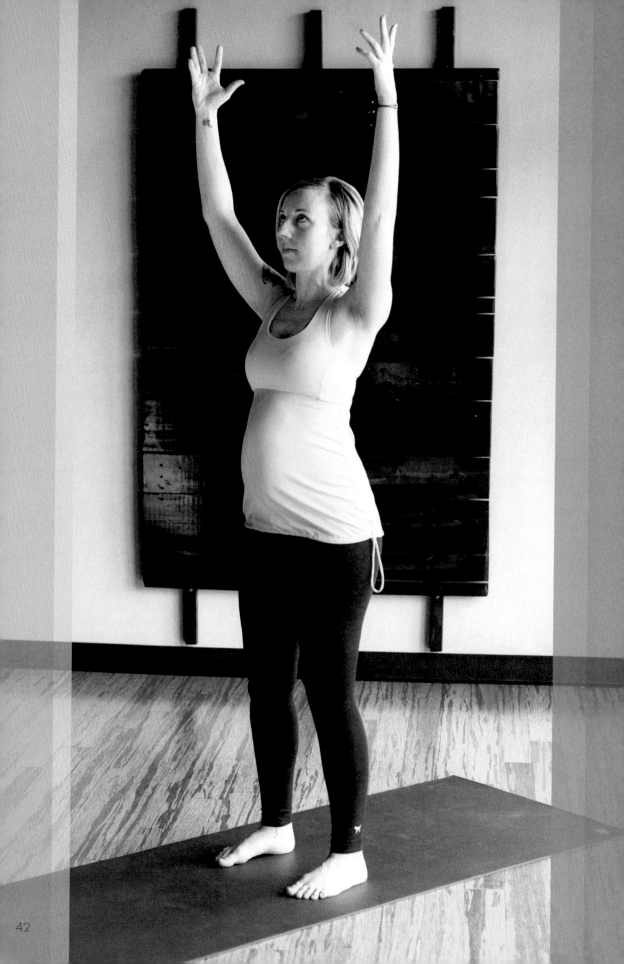

MOUNTAIN POSE

Slowly release to Mountain Pose, standing with your feet hip-width apart and your hands at the sides of your thighs, palms facing forward.

Feel the grounded, centering energy of the pose from the soles of your feet up through the crown of your head, and breathe into that feeling. — *four breaths here —*

Take a deep inhale, reaching your arms up to the sky, and as you exhale palms come together and to your heart center. Repeat with the following affirmations:

Inhale, "Trust in Birth" – with your exhale, draw it into your heart. Inhale, "Trust in Your Body" – with your exhale, draw that into your heart.

Inhale, reach up to the sky. As you exhale, bend your knees a lot, taking the feet wide, and fold forward. Inhale to a half-way lift with hands on shins, lengthening the spine – and as you exhale, slowly come down to hands and knees.

BENEFITS This pose is grounding and energizing, creating balance and stability in the body.

CHILD'S POSE

— four breaths —

Allow your head to melt back down onto your mat, take a deep inhale and open-up on the exhale, allowing all of the thoughts in your mind to fall out as you drop down deeper into your body with each breath.

reflections, clarifications &mementos

week 13

photos or momentos

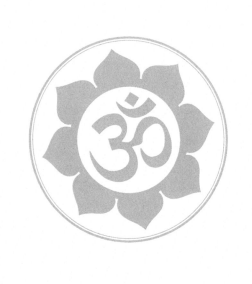

second
trimester
of pregnancy

M any women find the second trimester very enjoyable and exciting, as they are finally "showing" and can feel little flutters and movements from their growing baby.

The heavy fatigue and nausea of the first trimester decreases while energy levels are increasing, helping you enjoy what many women call the "Sweet Spot" of pregnancy.

By the end of the second trimester, your baby will be almost four times as big as it was at the end of the first trimester! Most women look forward to the 20-week ultrasound scan, when they get to "see" their baby while their care provider checks the baby's growth and development. Often parents look forward to finding out the sex of their baby during this scan.

SECOND TRIMESTER OF PREGNANCY AND YOGA

- After the first trimester of pregnancy, your care provider will encourage you to avoid lying on your back due to increased weight on the vena cava artery. Compression of the vena cava artery from the weight of your growing baby can result in feeling light-headed or having difficulty breathing due to a decrease in oxygen flow.

- If you are just beginning to practice yoga due to the newfound energy of the second trimester, take it slow and ease into completing the entire class.

YOGA POSES TO DISCONTINUE DURING THE SECOND TRIMESTER

- Chaturanga, Upward Dog

- Full Camel

- Wheel and any poses that create a similar feeling of pushing through the abdominal muscles

- Headstand and Handstand

- Any twist that does not include both "sit bones" on your mat

- Poses that include lying on your back for a prolonged period

- Arm balances

- Any pose that causes discomfort. Remember that as your baby grows, what felt good yesterday may feel very different today.

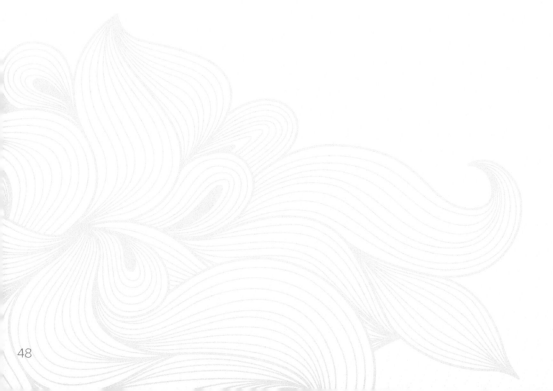

second trimester common ailments & birth wisdom yoga remedies

SPD (SYMPHYSIS PUBIS DYSFUNCTION)

Pubic Bone Pain caused by movement of the pelvis and ligaments around the pelvic area during pregnancy.

- Child's Pose with knees narrower than mat-width and room for your baby.
- Mountain Pose with feet hip-width apart and a micro-bend in the knees, palms facing forward and resting next to your thighs.
- Wall Plank with hands at shoulder height and pressing into the wall. Step feet back until it is easy to fold forward, soften the knees while moving the hips left and right.
- Hero's Pose with knees hip-width apart and a blanket in between feet.
- Bilateral Stretch from hands and knees, pressing right foot back and reaching forward with the left hand, then alternating sides.
- Cow and Cat poses.
- Chair Pose with block between thighs. Use the wall for support.
- Bridge Pose with block between thighs.
- Seated Twist with both sit bones on your mat. Walk the hands to the right and the left, gently reaching up and lengthening through your spine and the crown of your head.

DAILY TIPS FOR MINIMIZING SPD INFLAMMATION AND PAIN

- When you are getting in or out of a car, bed or bathtub, take extra care to keep your knees together as much as possible. If you are lying down, pull your knees up as far as you can before sitting up. This helps limit movement in the pelvis while making it easier to part your legs.
- When getting dressed in the morning, make sure you sit down to put on your pants.
- Slow down and listen to your body. If something hurts, if possible, don't repeat the movement that causes pain — because if it's allowed to flare up, it can take a long time to settle down again.
- Move often, but focus on small movements.
- When climbing stairs, take one step at a time. Step up onto one step with your best leg and then bring your other leg to meet it. Repeat with each step.
- In labor and childbirth, the hands and knees position with pelvic circles helps to minimize pain.

intuition

Learning to listen to your wisdom in pregnancy, birth and mothering is one of the challenges and great gifts of motherhood. When you become pregnant, you soon find there are various opinions about mothering – and people aren't afraid to share them! Slowing down and connecting to your breath will lead you to feeling your unique wisdom and intuition in each moment.

{affirmations}

*Through the practice of yoga, I am learning to
Pause, Breathe, and Feel what is best for my family.*

I close my eyes, going inside my body and out of my head.

*I am honored to go through labor and
bring my baby into the world.*

*I listen to my body, so I slow down, rest, and eat
when I need to replenish my energy.*

*I accept the Spiritual Birth of myself
from Woman to Mother.*

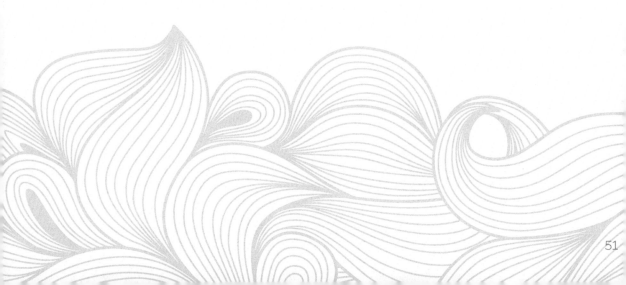

CREATING SACRED SPACE FOR YOU AND YOUR FAMILY

After a recent family vacation, I was reflecting on the gift of time with my family and the simplicity I enjoy when I am listening to and following my intuition. I find that it is very easy to get caught up in what I call "the frenzy" of making plans for vacation time and then to end up feeling worn out, rather than rejuvenated. As I prepared for our trip, I had to stop myself from making a list of things I wanted to share with my husband and children, and relax into feeling and listening versus planning.

Practicing what I speak about in Birth Wisdom Prenatal and Postpartum Yoga classes, and allowing our babies and children to lead the way, helps me to stay in the present moment and soak up authentic time with my family.

Nature, art and ritual have been at the core of our most sacred time together. Taking a nature walk and leaving our cell phones at home so we all can take in the smells, sounds and beauty of where we live, without the distraction of selfies and sharing, can be a deeply grounding experience for all of us. At home, taking out our paints and blank canvases and placing them on a utility table outside, inviting the children to paint whatever inspires them becomes a joyful, soul-soothing practice. The meditative art of creating, without fear or boundaries, is grounding and centering.

When the children were still in diapers, I would tape butcher paper to an easel outside and they would paint sheet after sheet — as many as they liked. The limitless amount of time and blank paper, combined with undirected time to create, led to my daughter asking for more white sheets of paper and pencils when she was a toddler. Often she would wake up in the morning with an idea in her mind as she burst down the hall to her big table (we never used the dining room table anyway). She would draw sheet after sheet of animals from her imagination, with old fashioned clothes and hats and stories to go along with them. The more room she had to draw, the calmer and more enjoyable she was at ages three, four and five. Now she is 15, and when I can tell she needs some grounding energy, I remind her to paint or draw. Most of the time she will start writing or drawing on her own after finishing her homework. I love knowing she has an endless, creative tool to get connected from her heart.

Drum circles became a fun ritual for the children when they were in preschool. Sitting in a circle with our drums, shakers and a "talking stick" adorned with ribbons and chimes, we shared drumming and reverence for sacred space. The children learned to speak only when they held the special "talking stick." With the passing of time, our circles organically flowed into celebrations for birthdays where we would light a candle and take turns drumming. I would hold the "Mother Goddess" drum, while passing our "Bear Drum" around the circle, each child taking a turn drumming with me. With the drum in their hands they would first express why they were grateful for their brother or sister who was celebrating his or her birthday, then drum with me until I stopped drumming. The Bear Drum would then be passed to the next child to share. Our circle also became a space to meet and pray if a child had a problem at school, or to hold a ceremony of gratitude for a "fallen guppy fish" we needed to say goodbye to.

Our drum circles became a beautiful, safe place to express love, fear or gratitude. The deep healing nature of our "Drum Circle Space" became even clearer in the Fall of 2010, when my daughter and I returned home to discover a robber in our home. Thankfully, upon our return he quickly fled out the back door and no one was injured. He did steal our best jewelry, computers, and the kids' piggy banks. Our house was turned upside down and everything had been picked through for valuables – even my son's clarinet had been taken apart and examined. The children were frightened that the robber would come back and would begin crying, even in the middle of the day, with fears of his return. I decided to hold a "fear releasing drum circle" ceremony. Each family member wrote on a piece of paper what he or she was afraid of in relation to the robber returning. My husband lit a fire in the fireplace, and we began our drum circle with a meditative prayer for each of us to let go of our fears. We each drummed one at a time, taking turns reading our fears out loud. Releasing them to the universe, we each threw our piece of paper with our fears into the fire. Then I spoke to my family about feeling what the young man must have been experiencing in his life, to risk going to jail for a long time by coming into our home and stealing our things. I asked them to think of what his life must be like, and to feel compassion for what he might have experienced that led him to steal from us. My husband then said a prayer for us all. The power of our sacred circle and ritual was confirmed by the children never expressing fear of the robber returning again. Learning compassion, even for someone who has hurt them, was a wonderful lesson of empathy and healing for the children at a very young age.

Nurturing myself by taking time to rejuvenate alone and with my husband, is vital to my ability to connect and stay present with our children during our daily lives. Sometimes, we believe we are too busy to take a moment for ourselves. Remembering the simplicity of what fills us up helps us find our path. A steaming bath is possible, even when your children are young. Water is deeply healing and cleansing, aiding in letting go of the energy of the day. Your partner will be motivated to take care of your little ones as he experiences the benefit of your connection together, after you have taken time to breathe and nurture yourself. Sometimes, as couples, we can feel overwhelmed by the moment-to-moment caring for our children – it feels like there is just not enough time for us to spend time alone together. Getting out of "the frenzy" of elaborate plans and date-nights by spending authentic time alone, can help create space for much-needed time to-gether. You may decide to wake up an hour earlier than usual to connect with each other before beginning your day, or even find your way to bed an hour earlier, rather than watching TV. These "stolen" moments add up to keeping you and your partner connected in a way that will fill you both up, rather than spending more busy-time that will wear you both out.

As you explore what fills you up as a woman, separate from your children or your spouse, I urge you to give yourself the gift of creating that space without guilt. I often hear moms express the mental and physical discom-fort of being away from their children. They explain that just as soon as they find time for themselves, they feel guilty for being away and have an urge to rush back home. I know I still feel that discomfort when my chil-dren are not with me, even though they are now 18, 15 and 12 years old. I have learned over time to teach our children that I need to love myself as much as I love them – and that part of that is creating space alone for me, and space alone with their Dad. When the children were younger, I would explain to them, "Mommy will be nicer if she goes to yoga," when I was desperate to get to a class alone and they wanted to come along.

It is natural and necessary for our connections with our children to run deep, but not at the expense of our love for ourselves or our partners. It takes practice to place ourselves at the top of the list. Remember that if we are nurtured and fed, our families will benefit from our calm, ground-ed and connected energy. We women set the tone for our entire families. Our power to create joyful and sacred space, for them and for ourselves, is endless.

reflections, clarifications &mementos

intuition

Where have you used your intuition this week to "feel about" an experience, rather than "think about" it?

_____

_____

_____

_____

_____

_____

Where in your life can you practice "opening up" to your wisdom and intuition before reacting?

_____

_____

_____

_____

_____

_____

What is coming up for you in meditation this week?

_____

_____

_____

Write a letter to your baby.

_____

_____

_____

_____

_____

_____

_____

_____

_____

_____

_____

_____

_____

photos or momentos

STEP-THROUGH TO WARRIOR POSES FROM HANDS AND KNEES

Take a deep inhale – and as you exhale, slowly move to hands and knees.

Bring your hands together, thumbs touching, with fingers wide and facing forward. This creates space so that, as your baby grows, you don't hit your belly with your knees.

Coming into **Warrior 1**: Step the left foot forward, press into right toes, drop the right heel down and, if needed, use the left thigh to come on up. Look back at your right foot: it should be slightly facing forward at a 45-degree angle, with right toes, knee and center of right hip facing the same direction. Soften the left knee.

Gently square the rib cage and shoulders forward, and reach up to the sky. Gently "hug" baby to spine to avoid over-arching. Shoulders melt down and away from your ears, biceps and fingers are strong. Soften the jaw and come into the breath completely.

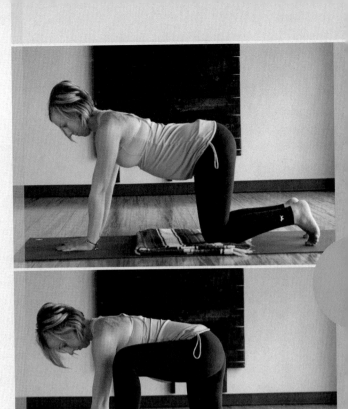

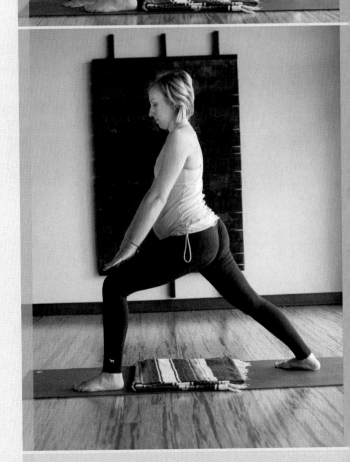

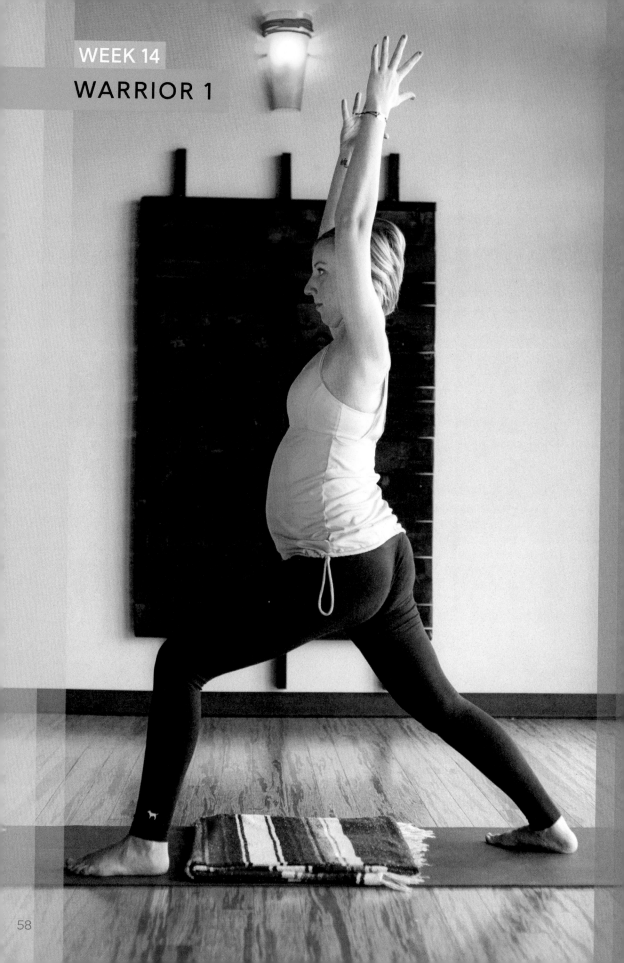

Breathe into your strength and power here. — *four breaths* —

BENEFITS Strengthens the legs, glutes and spine. Feeling your strength and power here is wonderful practice for the "marathon" of labor and childbirth.

MODIFICATIONS Inhale as you reach your hands up to the sky – on your exhale, softly straighten your left knee and allow your arms to flow behind you. Repeat four times with inhale, soften the left knee back down – and exhale, straightening the left knee with arms flowing back.

FLOWING DOWN TO YOUR MAT Take your left hand to your left thigh, drop the right knee and right hand to your mat, returning to hands and knees.

PRENATAL CHATURANGA For Prenatal Chaturanga you have options. You can come to Child's Pose, five Mini-Push-Ups, Pelvic Circles, Cow & Cat or Downward Facing Dog. You decide what feels good in your body. What do you need to feel strong while also taking care of yourself here?

— *five breaths* —

●●● **STEP THROUGH TO WARRIOR 1 RIGHT SIDE** Take a deep inhale – and as you exhale, slowly move to hands and knees. Bringing your hands together in the center of your mat, thumbs touching and fingers facing forward, step the right foot forward, press into left toes, drop the left heel down, and use the right thigh if needed to come on up.

Breathe into your strength and power here. — *four breaths* —

FLOWING DOWN TO YOUR MAT Take your right hand to your right thigh, drop the left knee and left hand to your mat, returning to hands and knees.

PRENATAL CHATURANGA For Prenatal Chaturanga you have options. You can come to Child's Pose, five Mini-Push-Ups, Pelvic Circles, Cow & Cat or Downward Facing Dog. You decide what feels good in your body. What do you need to feel strong while also taking care of yourself here?

— *five breaths* —

Downward Facing Dog or Child's Pose. — *four breaths* —

reflections, clarifications &mementos

week 14

photos or momentos

PRENATAL CHATURANGA

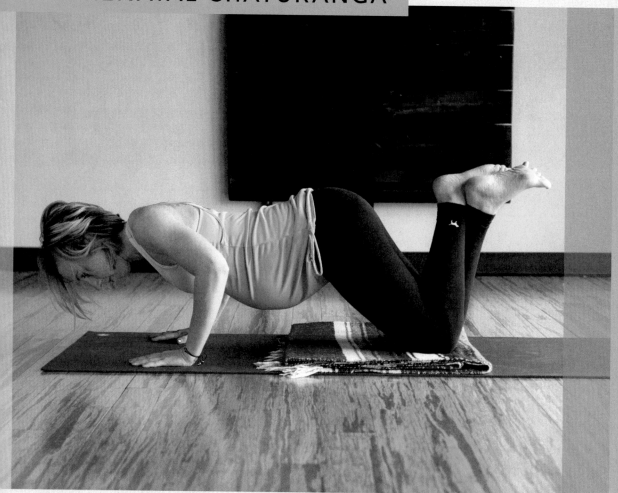

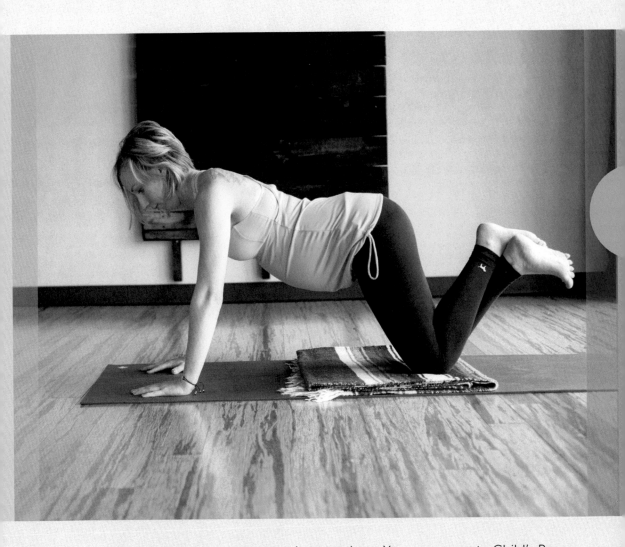

For Prenatal Chaturanga you have options. You can come to Child's Pose, five Mini-Push-Ups, Pelvic Circles, Cow & Cat or Downward Facing Dog. You decide what feels good in your body. What do you need to feel strong while also taking care of yourself here? — *five breaths* —

BENEFITS Strengthens the upper body while allowing space to reconnect to the breath when needed.

reflections, clarifications & mementos

week 15

photos or momentos

65

WARRIOR 2

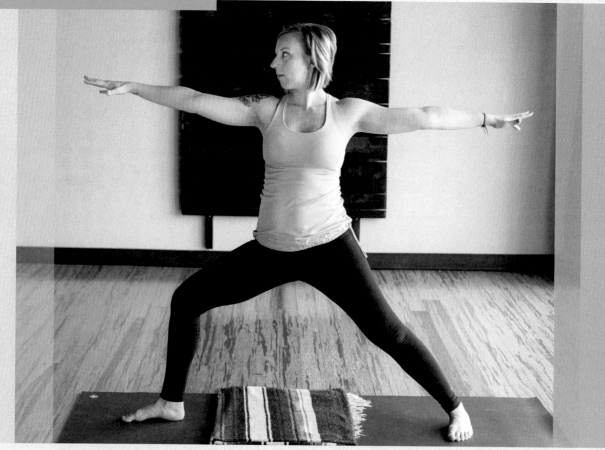

SETTING UP FOR WARRIOR 2

From hands and knees, bring your hands together in the center of your mat, thumbs touching and fingers facing forward. Step the right foot forward, plant the left foot all the way down, with left toes facing the left side of your mat, using the right thigh to come up if needed. Your right heel is lined up with the inside of your left arch, adjusting where it feels good for you. Gently square the hips and shoulders to the left side of your mat, right hand forward, left hand back, soften the shoulders down and away from the ears, with your gaze forward and over the right fingertips. Feel the line of energy from your right fingertips, across your shoulder blades and into your left fingertips. Breathe into it. — *four breaths* —

BENEFITS Strengthens the legs, glutes and spine. Feel your strength and power here. This pose is wonderful practice for the "marathon" of labor and childbirth. Gently strengthens the arms, legs, and core.

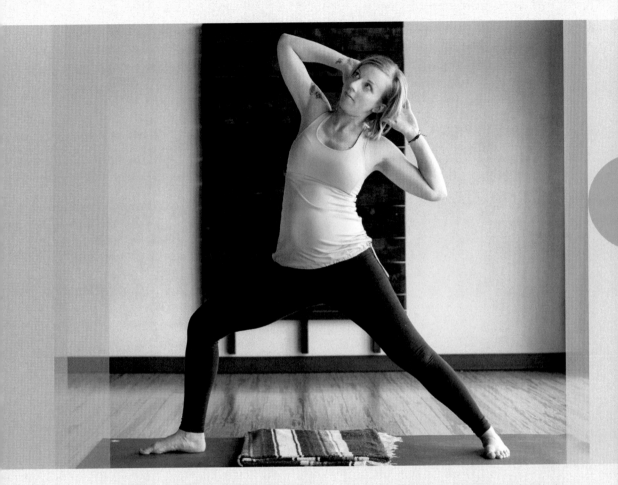

MODIFICATION FOR WARRIOR 2 If you want to take the pose a little deeper, bring your hands behind your head, slowly rocking your elbows to the sky with your breath. You will feel the micro-muscles of your inner thighs waking up here.

FLOWING DOWN TO YOUR MAT FROM WARRIOR 2 Take your right hand to your right thigh, drop the left knee and left hand to your mat, returning to hands and knees.

PRENATAL CHATURANGA For Prenatal Chaturanga you have options. You can come to Child's Pose, five Mini-Push-Ups, Pelvic Circles, Cow & Cat or Downward Facing Dog. You decide what feels good in your body. What do you need to feel strong while also taking care of yourself here?
— *five breaths* —

Downward Facing Dog or Child's Pose. — *four breaths* —

Deep inhale – as you exhale, flow down to hands and knees.

reflections, clarifications &mementos

week 16

photos or momentos

surrender

There comes a point in every woman's labor when surrendering to the sensations she is feeling will help her labor progress. It is important to remember that if our contractions don't get stronger and closer together, we cannot birth our babies. With an attitude of acceptance and surrender, we can welcome each wave of contractions. Asking for more and diving into the contractions is an empowering state of mind. Focus on releasing each contraction with a thank you, while softening your body completely until the next wave begins.

We can approach challenges in our lives with acceptance and surrender as well. As we practice surrendering to challenges and choosing to trust rather than resist, our experiences will transform. We benefit from the gift of "pearls of wisdom" in even our most difficult life experiences.

{affirmations}

I am learning to Surrender into each moment
of this pregnancy, allowing my baby to lead the way,
just as I will in motherhood.

I let go of all rigid ideas of our birth experience,
and I replace them with an open mind for the "Adventure of Birth."
I have intentions for our birthing experience, and
I recognize that surrendering to labor begins now.

During labor and childbirth, I intend to Surrender to my body,
welcoming each contraction and diving into the sensations I feel,
knowing it is the way to my baby.

I stay focused, riding each wave of contractions like water.
I am soft, I am fluid.

I release each contraction as I exhale,
saying thank you for creating space for my baby.

REMEMBER THE CHEERIO

For years, I struggled with the "messiness" of mothering. Each night, after all three children were in bed, I would walk through the house and attempt to put everything in its place. Most importantly, I would take toys that had made their way into my bedroom and put them out of sight. It would give me a feeling of peace and room to breathe, like I was reclaiming my space.

One night, I had finished my ritual of cleaning, and everything was in order. With candles lit and my favorite book, I happily slipped into a steaming, hot tub. Perfection! As I relaxed into the water and exhaled from another hectic day, I glimpsed something floating by. I scooped it out of the water and realized I was not the only thing steaming in the tub – it was a Cheerio! I took the soggy Cheerio out of the tub, and set it on the tile. Gazing at the water-logged piece of cereal, I realized the "messiness" of motherhood was never going to leave me. I wondered: In my attempt to make everything look perfect, was I missing out on the good stuff?

I began to realize that in "surrendering to the mess" of everyday mothering, I could find the space to relax into the experience of motherhood on a deeper level. When I am distracted with perfection as a mother, I lose sight of the beauty and joy of my daily life. My calling as a mother is not to have the perfect house, car, or children. My calling is to let go of society's perceptions of what a "perfect" family looks like, and surrender to the beauty of mothering my children authentically – despite how it might look in the moment.

Today, I see the "little messes" in our home as symbols of our children still being here with us. Someday, my house will be "perfect" again, with no sign of children running through it – and I will be wishing for those little fingerprints on the walls, and the sounds of squealing toddlers racing down the halls.

BIRTH WISDOM FOUR

reflections, clarifications &mementos

surrender

Where can you practice surrendering to ***what is*** *during this pregnancy?*

What does surrendering in labor and childbirth mean to you?

What is coming up for you in meditation this week?

Write a letter to your baby.

_____

_____

_____

_____

_____

_____

_____

_____

_____

_____

_____

_____

_____

photos or momentos

TRIANGLE POSE

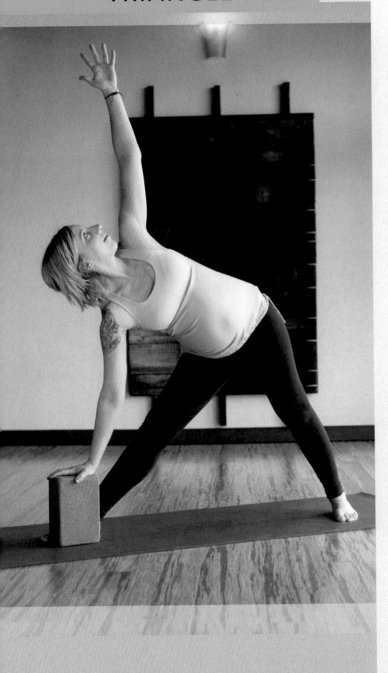

TRANSITION TO TRIANGLE POSE FROM WARRIOR 2 RIGHT SIDE

From hands and knees, bring your hands together in the center of your mat, thumbs touching and fingers facing forward. Step the right foot forward and left foot down, using the right thigh if needed to come on up to Warrior 2.

Inhale, reach the right hand forward and straighten the right leg, keeping a micro-bend in the knee – and with your block in front of your right ankle, open your arms into triangle pose.

Right hand rests on your block for support as left hand reaches to the sky, opening your heart.
— *four breaths* —

BENEFITS Tones and lengthens the muscles of the pelvic floor, building strength for pushing in labor. Creates strength and balance in the legs, spine and arms.

reflections, clarifications &mementos

week 17

photos or momentos

REVERSE WARRIOR

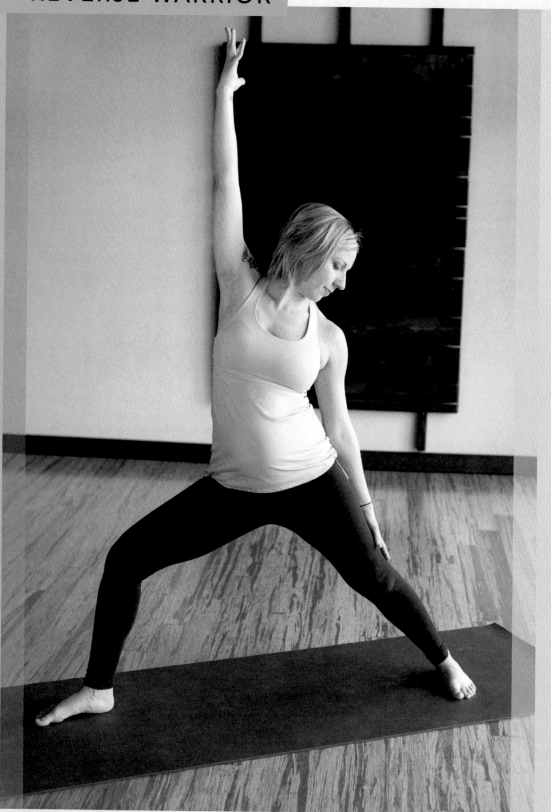

TRANSITION TO REVERSE WARRIOR
FROM TRIANGLE POSE RIGHT SIDE

From Triangle Pose take a deep inhale – and as you exhale, bend the right knee gently while taking your left hand down and your right hand to the sky. — *four breaths* —

BENEFITS Opens up the side of the body, while strengthening the legs.

FLOWING BACK DOWN TO YOUR MAT Take your right hand to your right thigh, drop your left knee and left hand to the mat, and return to hands and knees.

PRENATAL CHATURANGA For Prenatal Chaturanga you have options. You can come to Child's Pose, five Mini-Push-Ups, Pelvic Circles, Cow & Cat or Downward Facing Dog. You decide what feels good in your body. What do you need to feel strong while also taking care of yourself here?
— *five breaths* —

Repeat Triangle Pose and Reverse Warrior Left Side

PRENATAL CHATURANGA For Prenatal Chaturanga you have options. You can come to Child's Pose, five Mini-Push-Ups, Pelvic Circles, Cow & Cat or Downward Facing Dog. You decide what feels good in your body. What do you need to feel strong while also taking care of yourself here?
— *five breaths* —

Downward Facing Dog or Child's Pose. — *three breaths* —

Deep inhale – as you exhale, move to Downward Facing Dog if not already there.

reflections, clarifications &mementos

photos or moments

GODDESS POSE

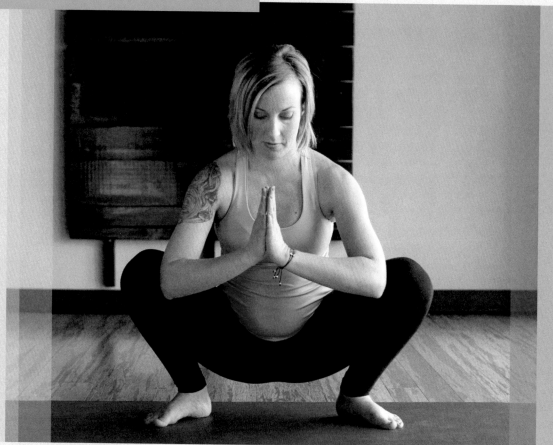

From Downward Facing Dog, take a deep inhale – and as you exhale, bend your knees a lot and walk your hands back toward your feet, step your feet out to the sides of your mat with toes pointing out, coming into Goddess Pose. Bring your palms together at heart-center, and breathe. Soften the jaw, and allow the shoulders to melt down away from your ears. Breathe here for up to one minute, about the length of a contraction. Use your breath to go deep inside.

Remember, contractions are like waves in the ocean: They go up and always come down. You only need to breathe to the top of each wave, and then each contraction releases. See if you can notice the sensations in your body here and dive into what you are feeling. If you need to sit on a block for support, go there. If you are feeling strong, stay with it for five more breaths. Inhale deep – and as you exhale, slowly release to hands and knees. Arch your back into Cat Pose, curl your toes, and find your way into Downward Facing Dog.

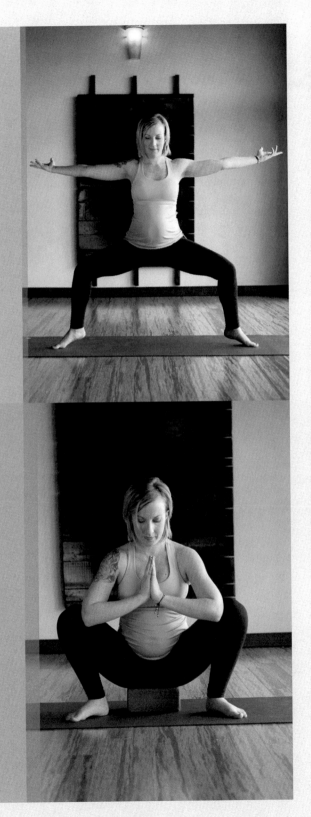

MODIFICATIONS FOR GODDESS POSE

If you want to take it deeper, come into a wide-leg Goddess Pose and lift the heels. — *three to five breaths* —

If your heels do not touch your mat while in Goddess Pose, use a block on the lowest setting to find support and ease with your breath.

BENEFITS Wonderful preparation for labor and childbirth. This pose is often used and recommended for the pushing stage of labor. Opens the pelvic outlet and creates space for baby in birth. Lengthens and strengthens the pelvic floor muscles, legs and glutes.

PRENATAL CHATURANGA From Goddess Pose, release to hands and knees. You can come to Child's Pose, five Mini-Push-Ups, Pelvic Circles, Cow & Cat or Downward Facing Dog. You decide what feels good in your body. What do you need to feel strong while also taking care of yourself? — *five breaths* —

Downward Facing Dog or Child's Pose. — *three breaths* —

reflections, clarifications & mementos

week 19

photos or momentos

GODDESS STRETCHES

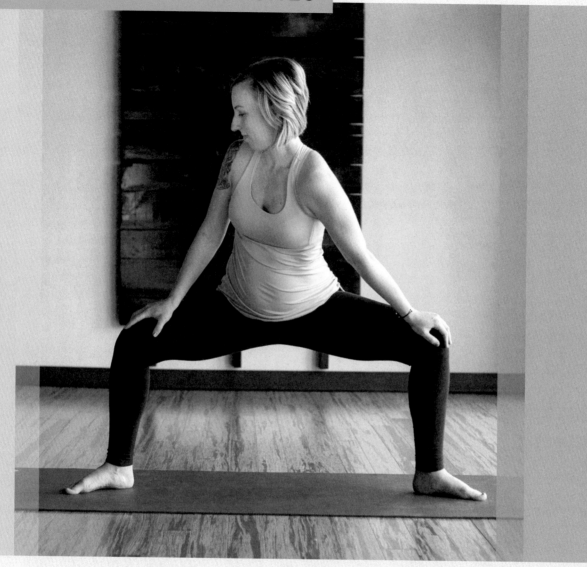

From Downward Facing Dog, bend your knees deeply, walk your hands to your feet, and slowly stand up. Standing in a wide goddess pose, place your right hand on your right thigh, and your left hand on your left thigh, turning your head from the left to right while alternating pressing your hands into your left and right thighs, opening up your spine.

To take the stretch deeper, place a block in front of you, gently folding forward while placing one hand on your block and reaching the opposite hand up to the sky. Alternate with your breath, inhaling to the sky and exhaling down to your block.

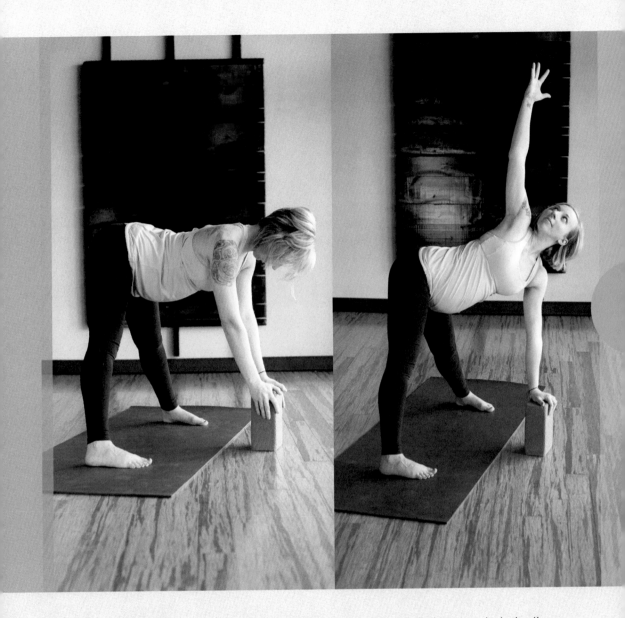

BENEFITS Creates space in the rib cage and can help move baby's elbows or feet out of mom's ribs. Stretches and opens up the spine, ribcage and legs.

PRENATAL CHATURANGA From Wide Goddess Pose, release to hands and knees. You can come to Child's Pose, five Mini-Push-Ups, Pelvic Circles, Cow & Cat or Downward Facing Dog. You decide what feels good in your body. What do you need to feel strong while also taking care of yourself here? — *five breaths* —

Downward Facing Dog or Child's Pose. — *three breaths* —

reflections, clarifications &mementos

week 20

photos or moments

trust birth

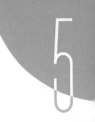

> Tonight in class, Julia, you said something that really resonated with me — that "worrying is the work of pregnancy"[1] — and we worked on letting go of worry and relying on our own strength, both in discussion and by practicing our breathing. I had been mulling over a similar quote all day from Mark Twain: "I've had a lot of worries in my life, most of which never happened."
>
> Thank you for acknowledging that worry is a common theme for pregnant women and re-affirming that our own innate strength and wisdom can be trusted and honored wherever our birthing path takes us. We can use that worry to ask questions, so that we can find answers. And it is with that knowledge that we gain confidence. *– Rachel, Birth Wisdom Yoga prenatal and postpartum student*

Trusting that our lives are guided by a source of positive energy helps to release resistance and fear. When we know that we are right where we are meant to be in every moment, we are free of negative thoughts that do not serve us well. Whenever you are feeling drained and tired, ask yourself what it is that you are resisting. Trusting that our path is guided by divine love and perfect abundance opens us up to endless possibilities in pregnancy, childbirth and mothering.

{affirmations}

I see my baby feeling secure, safe and surrounded by a bright, glowing light of serenity and protection.

I know that we will receive the wisdom, patience and understanding that we need as parents. I trust our instincts to know what our baby needs and to let go of worries about the future.

I am full of gratitude for my body, and for the beautiful rhythm of my baby leading the way, my body following wisely.

---

[1] *Birthing From Within*, England & Horowitz

DIASTASIS RECTI AND PRENATAL YOGA

Diastasis Recti is caused by the amount of pressure on the abdominal muscles during pregnancy. *Diastasis* means separation. *Recti* refers to the abdominal muscle, the *rectus abdominis*. When the muscles of the left and right side of the abdomen widen due to pregnancy, the bowels, uterus and other major organs have only a thin band of connective tissue to support them in place. Common yoga and abdominal exercises practiced prenatally and postpartum, can make a *diastasis recti* worse when not modified.

Poses to discontinue while pregnant and until at least four months postpartum, to ensure optimal healing of the abdominal muscles include:

- Low Cobra
- Up Dog
- High Plank and Forearm Plank if you have a Diastasis of 3-4 inches. Consult a Physical Therapist for guidelines on when to resume Plank poses.
- Wheel
- Locust
- Full Camel
- Bow
- Anything that creates a feeling of "pushing open the abs."

BIRTH WISDOM FIVE

reflections, clarifications &mementos

trust birth

What worries do you feel that you can explore and find answers to?

Is there anything that you are resisting that you can use Trust to let go of?

What is coming up for you in meditation this week?

Write a letter to your baby.

photos or momentos

GATE POSE

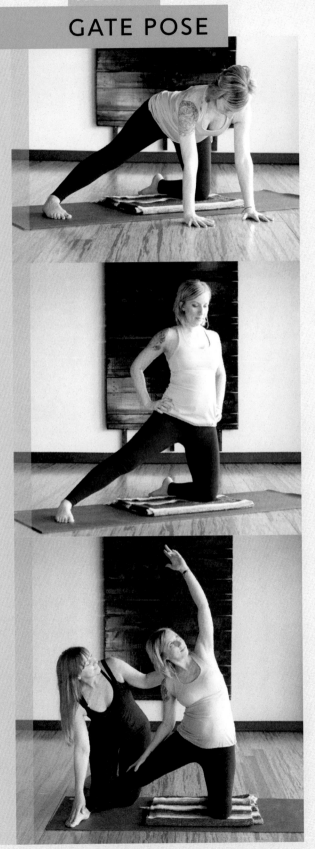

Slowly come down to hands and knees. Still facing the side of your mat, press into your hands and step the right foot out to the side. Find stability first, then take your hands up to your hips and slide your right hand down your right thigh as your left hand reaches to the sky.

— four breaths —

Come back to hands and knees, and slowly change sides. Press into your hands, step the left foot out to the side, take your hands up to your hips, and slide the left hand down the left thigh as your right hand reaches to the sky.

— four breaths —

Slowly come back to hands and knees. Arch your back, curl your toes and press back into Downward Facing Dog. Deep inhale, deep exhale. Inhale – and as you exhale, bend your knees deeply and walk your hands back to your feet, slowly standing up.

BENEFITS Strengthens and lengthens the muscles and ligaments of the pelvic floor. Strengthens the inner thighs and calves.

reflections, clarifications &mementos

week 21

photos or momentos

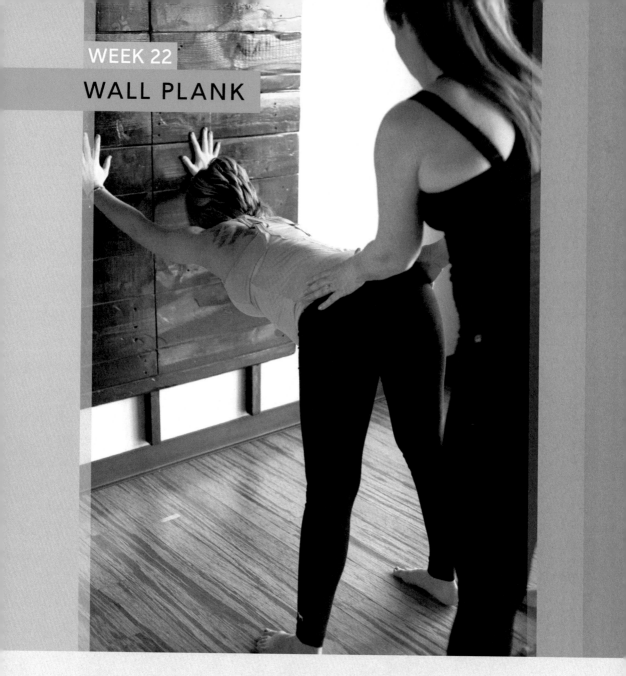

WEEK 22
WALL PLANK

Standing, with your palms pressing into the wall at shoulder height, walk your feet back wide and drop your head. Lengthen the spine, move the hips left and right while softening the knees. — *five breaths* —

BENEFITS Releases and opens up the lower back, arms and shoulders. In labor and childbirth, gives birth partner access to mom's lower back for counter-pressure pain relief and opens up the pelvic outlet, creating space for baby.

reflections, clarifications &mementos

week 22

photos or momentos

SLOW DANCING

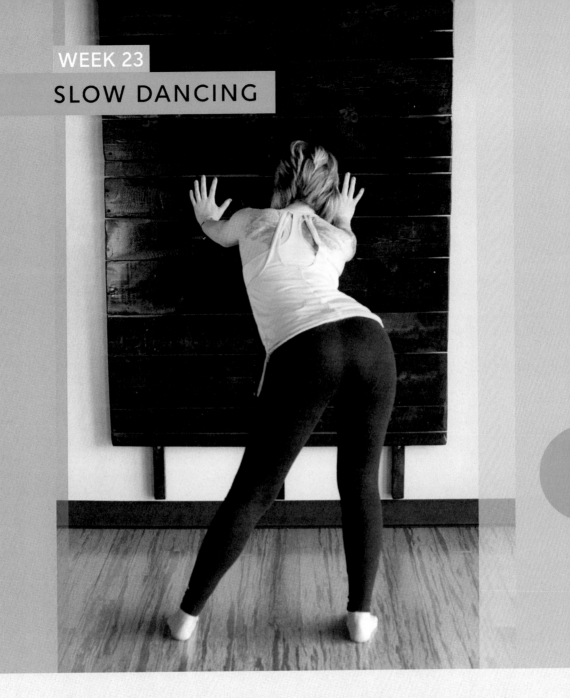

Taking a few steps closer to the wall, come into pelvic circles to the right and left with knees soft. Move where it feels good for you, while releasing the hips and lower back completely. — *five breaths* —

BENEFITS This is an optimal position for early and active labor. Use your birth partner or the wall for support. With the feet nice and wide, this pose creates space for your baby while gravity is working for you. During labor, alternate with walking to create a rhythm with the breath, which many women describe as their "lifeline" in labor and childbirth.

reflections, clarifications &mementos

photos or momentos

103

HALF MOON POSE ON THE WALL

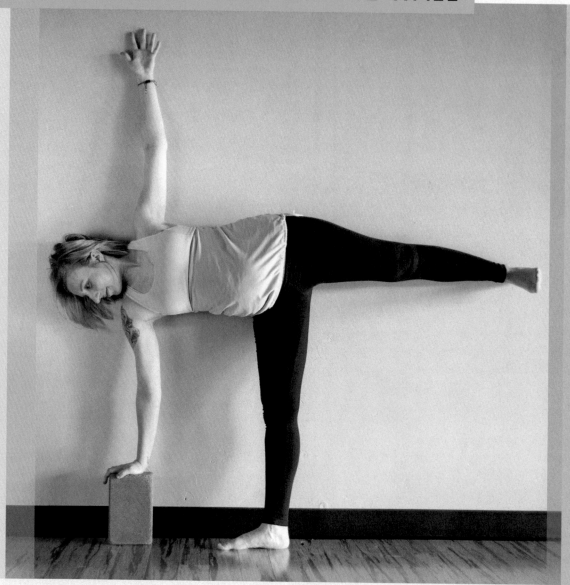

Placing a block in front of your right foot, directly under your right shoulder, press down with your right hand while lifting your left hand to the sky and your left leg in line with your left hip, or lower. Allow the left hip and left shoulder to roll into the wall for support. — *five breaths* —

Repeat on left side.

BENEFITS Completely releases the ligaments on each side of the body, while helping to remedy sciatic pain. Women who are close to full-term or carrying twins will often enjoy the release of this pose.

reflections, clarifications &mementos

week 24

photos or momentos

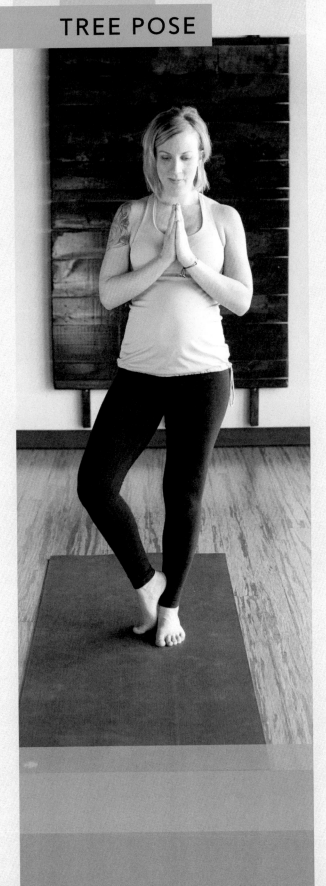

TREE POSE

Pressing down into your left foot, feel your heel and the edges of your left foot on your mat. Take a micro-bend in your left knee for stability. Begin by placing your right foot next to your left ankle, and find your breath.

It is more beneficial when you are pregnant to practice a modified tree pose, which creates balance in the body, rather than using the wall to balance and taking the free leg higher.

If it feels good for you to take the free leg higher, place your hands on your hips for stability and lift your right foot up and below the left knee.

If you would like a deeper pose, place your right leg above your left knee, with hands reaching up to the sky.

— three to five breaths —

BENEFITS Creates balance and energy in the body. This is where your body can adjust to the changes in the pelvis due to pregnancy that create instability, finding balance again.

Tree pose is a wonderful reminder of how serious we can become when we "fall out" of the pose and need to begin again. We can practice being gentle with ourselves here and take that self-love into our mothering. Remembering to love ourselves even when we "fall out of it" (whatever the "it" is), knowing we can use our breath and begin again.

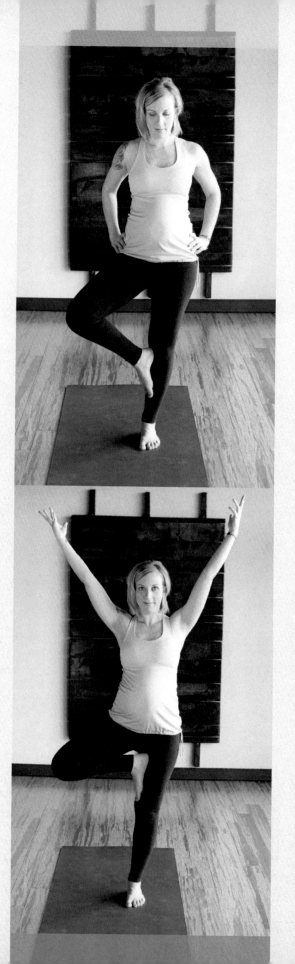

reflections, clarifications &mementos

week 25

photos or momentos

softening

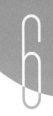

We practice "Birth Wisdom Yoga Softening" in Birth Wisdom Prenatal Yoga classes to prepare for the "resting period" you will have in between contractions. The more you can relax and soften your body between contractions, the faster your body can open up with less pain. Breathing through the contractions and softening in-between contractions creates a rhythm in labor that for many women becomes their "lifeline" for staying on top of the pain.

The ability to soften into **what is** is a gift of feminine energy that will serve you in childbirth and your daily life. When you can embrace your feminine powers — such as intuition, emotional connection and fluidity — you will be standing in your full power. Breath, stillness and journaling can help you embrace your feminine gifts and strengths with clarity.

Today, notice if you can allow yourself to "soften" into this experience of pregnancy, allowing this new version of self mentally and physically, to become a celebration of Women's Wisdom.

─────────{affirmations}─────────

With each Breath, I soften into my Divine Feminine Power and Strength, connecting to compassion for myself and my "sisters in motherhood."

I allow the edges of my entire body to soften like warm wax dripping down a candle.

In my ability to soften my entire body in between contractions, I open and dilate perfectly, diving into my Birthing Power and creating my own rhythm and focal point for labor and childbirth.

BIRTH WISDOM YOGA SOFTENING

Birth Wisdom Yoga Softening is a relaxation technique practiced in Birth Wisdom Prenatal Yoga classes. Combining the breath with Yin Yoga poses such as Butterfly, Pigeon, Seated Straddle, Supta Bhada Konasana or Child's Pose with visualization, will help you prepare for labor and childbirth.

This is what it looks like: Settling into the pose of your choice, allow your eyes to shut down and take a deep inhale all the way up to the sky. With your exhale, open your mouth and sigh everything out. Beginning with the crown of your head, slowly scan your body for tension, resistance, and even pain, taking your breath there and softening completely. Picture the edges of your body slowly "melting away" like warm wax from a candle. Continue to soften your entire body until you reach your toes.

This is what it looks like in labor and childbirth:

- Contraction begins. Take a deep cleansing breath, inhale all the way up through the crown of your head – and on your exhale let everything go, breathing all the way down and out your toes. Continue your Birth Wisdom Yoga Breathing, long and slow breaths all the way to the top of each contraction. Remember, contractions are like waves in the ocean: They always go up, and they always come down. You only need to focus on breathing to the top of each contraction, knowing that it will eventually release.

- As the contraction releases, gently soften your shoulders so they move away from your ears, and take a deep cleansing breath, saying thank you and letting that contraction go completely. Soften your jaw and release your fingers and toes. Breathe into how good it feels to let go of that contraction.

- Once the contraction ends, you will have a "resting period" of a few minutes. This "resting period" gets shorter as your baby is closer to being born. During this time, begin to "scan" your entire body, beginning with the crown of your head and notice where there is tension or resistance – and take your breath there, softening completely for your baby. Relax your jaw and picture the edges of your body melting away.

- This is a powerful technique that will help you go deep inside, find your focal point in labor with the breath, and stay on top of the contractions.

BIRTH WISDOM SIX

reflections, clarifications & mementos

softening

*Where can you soften into **what is** in your everyday life, embracing your feminine powers of intuition, emotional connection and fluidity?*

Do you find softening into this experience of pregnancy and this new version of self mentally and physically inspiring, challenging, or both?

What is coming up for you in meditation this week?

Write a letter to your baby.

photos or mementos

BUTTERFLY POSE

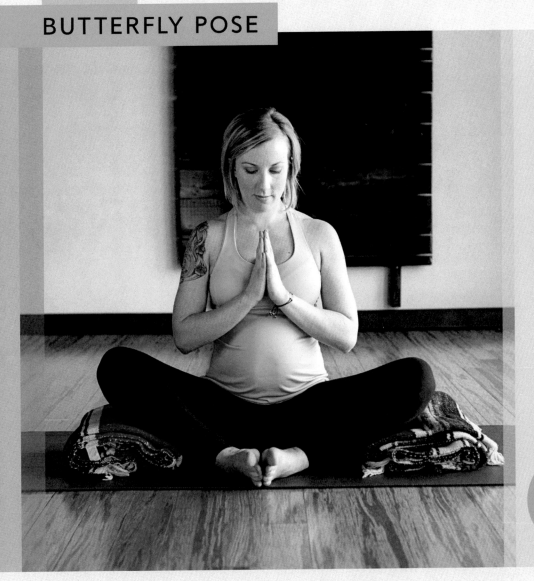

In a seated position, with a blanket underneath you for comfort if needed, bring the soles of the feet together. With a block under each thigh for support, sit up tall in the spine and take a deep cleansing breath, inhaling up to the sky and exhaling down and out your toes. — *five breaths* —

BENEFITS Encourages blood flow to the hips while opening the pelvic outlet. Creates space for baby to engage in the pelvis the last few weeks of pregnancy.

MODIFICATIONS If you are in the last weeks of pregnancy and know your baby is in a Breech position, you will not take this pose due to its ability to help baby engage into the pelvis.

reflections, clarifications & mementos

week 26

photos or momentos

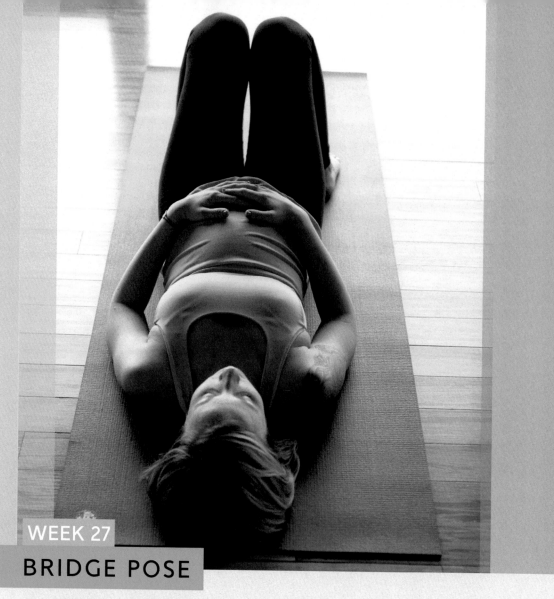

BRIDGE POSE

LEG CRAMPS AND PREGNANCY

It is very common to experience leg cramps during pregnancy due to additional weight gained and changes in your circulation. Most often, these cramps occur at night while sleeping. A very helpful way to release the pain is to come into Bridge Pose as soon as you feel a cramp beginning. Students report this remedy brings immediate relief from the pain associated with leg cramps.

Lie on your back with two blankets placed under your spine from your sacrum to your shoulders. If you are experiencing SPD or pubic bone pain, keep knees closer together as shown here. If not, place feet hip-width apart with heels under your knees. Press through your heels while using your legs to lift your hips up towards the sky. Hold for four-five breaths, then slowly release. Repeat as needed.

reflections, clarifications &mementos

week 27

photos or momentos

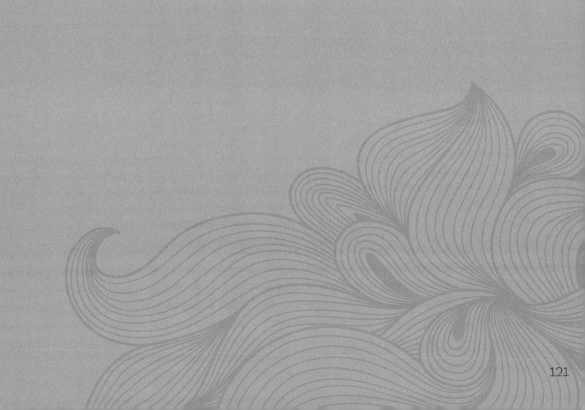

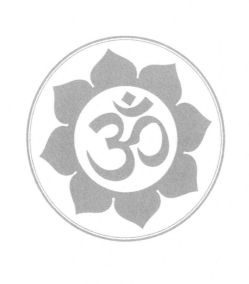
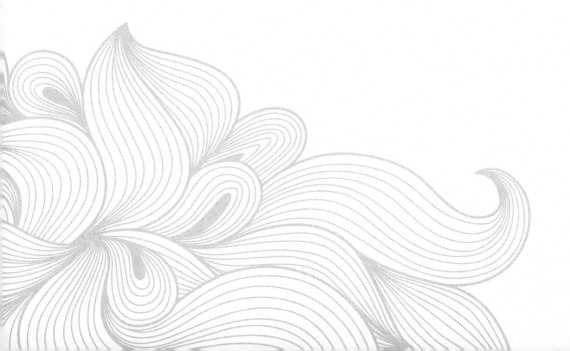

third
trimester
of pregnancy

WEEKS 28 TO 40+

The Third Trimester can be challenging as the fatigue that you felt in the first trimester often returns, alternating with bursts of energy that lead to "nesting" and organizing, followed by a feeling the next day that you may have "overdone it." This is a good time to pace yourself no matter how intense those "nesting" urges are! Sleep can become more of a challenge, because back and hip soreness may deepen and frequent urination returns. Listening to your body is essential to get the rest you need.

Appointments with your healthcare provider will increase to every two weeks during this time. Your OB or Midwife will also check to determine the position of your baby. This is often a time of focus on birth preparation and child birthing classes.

The frequent kicks and movement of your baby are an exciting reminder that it won't be long before you are holding him or her in your arms!

THIRD TRIMESTER OF PREGNANCY AND YOGA

- Listen to your body, and take Child's Pose or Easy Seated Position with the breath, as needed.

- Create space for your baby in Forward Folds, by taking the feet nice and wide with bent knees.

- Use a block under your forehead to create space in Child's Pose.

- Your yoga mat is your space to nurture yourself and do what feels good in your body. With each pose you are practicing for labor and childbirth while using the breath to stay in the present moment.

YOGA POSES TO DISCONTINUE DURING THE THIRD TRIMESTER

- Downward Facing Dog is often replaced with Hands and Knees Pose or Pelvic Circles for comfort. Standing and using the wall with hands placed at shoulder height and finding Pelvic Circles is also a welcome modification. If it feels good, continue practicing Downward Facing Dog.

- Discontinue Downward Facing Dog if your baby was in a breech position during the last few weeks of pregnancy, and was manually turned into a head-down position by your OB.

- If you are feeling low blood sugar or dizziness, discontinue Downward Facing Dog.

THIRD TRIMESTER MODIFICATIONS

- Bilateral Stretch:
  Keep toes of extended leg behind you on your mat to protect the ligaments and muscles in the lower back, groin, hips and pelvis.

- Warrior Series Poses:
  As your baby grows, it is important to shorten your stance and take your feet wider in warrior poses for stability.

- Warrior 1:
  Feet are hip-width apart and come closer together.

- Hug your baby gently to your spine in all standing poses to protect your lower back and decrease lower back pain.

- Goddess Pose with or without a block for support.

third trimester common ailments & birth wisdom yoga remedies

BREECH POSITIONED BABY

- Birth Wisdom Yoga Hands and Knees sequence, including Pelvic Circles, opens the pelvic floor outlet and encourages baby to turn.

- Supported Bridge with a block, placing the block standing tall, so head to hip ratio is 45°, two or three times a day. Alternate with Rocking Happy Baby Pose.

- Downward Facing Dog. Four breaths at a time.

- Standing Pelvic Circles, using the wall for support.

- Table Top Extension from hands and knees: step right foot out to the side and come slowly into Pelvic Circles. Change sides.

- Visualization of your baby turning into a head-down position while in these poses can be very effective.

- Acupressure Points. Acupressure can be very helpful for turning breech positioned babies. Find a doctor of Acupressure and/or Acupuncture in your area who specializes in pregnancy, rather than attempting to find the pressure points yourself.

- Chiropractic can be very helpful – particularly a doctor that specializes in the Webster Technique, which aligns the pelvis, helping breech positioned babies turn.

- Additional support can be found on the following website: www.spinningbabies.com.

- Once baby is head down, practice Bound Angle Pose or Butterfly Pose with the soles of your feet together and knees out wide, to help baby's head engage in the pelvis. (This pose is to be avoided while baby is still in a breech position.)

letting go

MEDITATION FOR LETTING GO

In a seated position, come into your breath. Allow your inhale to reach up to the sky – and your exhale to move down, around your baby and out your toes. Soften your jaw and allow your shoulders to melt down away from your ears. Picture a beautiful crystal at the base of your sit bones, connecting you and grounding you to the earth. See the beautiful golden light surrounding your entire body. Your energy field is a vibrant golden light surrounding you in love and protection, attracting abundance and health. See that golden light surrounding your baby completely. Breathe into knowing that your baby is so peaceful and content, right here inside of you. Breathe here for five minutes.

From this grounded and protected space, ask yourself what one thing you can let go of that is no longer serving you. It may be a worry, an emotion or an experience. It's usually the first thing that comes into your mind. Allow yourself to see what it looks like completely and feel what it feels like. As you breathe and exhale, begin to allow whatever it is to float back out to the universe. Say thank you and release with the breath, until it is on the other side of your energy field. Let it go with love and gratitude. Breathe here for five minutes. You can continue letting go of whatever it is that is no longer serving you. As you move through your daily life, with each exhale continue to release and let go.

———————— {affirmations} ————————

I am learning to let go now, just as I will in motherhood.
I allow my baby to lead the way.

I have completely surrendered to my body.
I trust, with gratitude, the good work my body is doing
to grow and sustain my baby.

As a woman, I have the unlimited power to birth my baby in
harmony with my baby's rhythm; I let her/him lead the way.

BIRTH WISDOM SEVEN

reflections, clarifications & mementos

letting go

What can you let go of this week that is no longer serving you?

What does "allowing your baby to lead the way" mean to you in pregnancy and childbirth?

What is coming up for you in meditation this week?

Write a letter to your baby.

_____

_____

_____

_____

_____

_____

_____

_____

_____

_____

_____

_____

photos or momentos

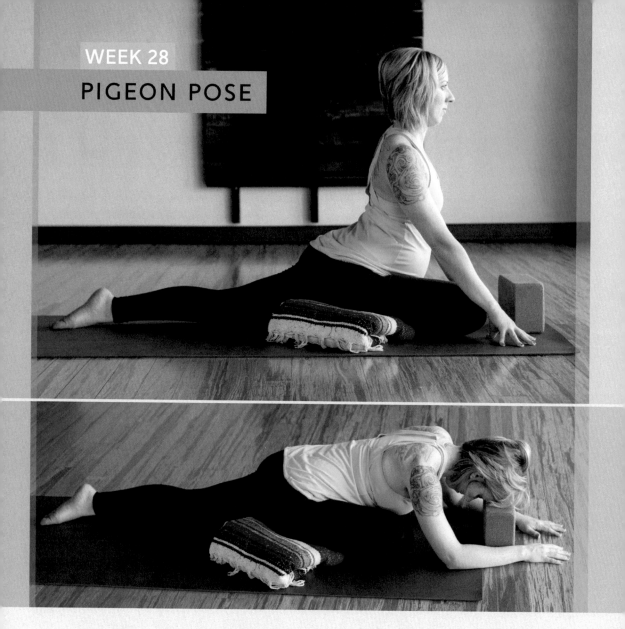

PIGEON POSE

From hands and knees, extend your right leg behind you and then gently bring the right knee forward towards the middle of your hands. Allow your right foot to soften down with your hips gently squared toward the top of your mat. Extend the left leg back behind you, or soften the knee if needed. Place a blanket under the right hip for support and a block in front of you on the high or low setting to create space for your baby. Inhale as you lengthen the spine – with your exhale, fold forward. — *five breaths* — Practice your Birth Wisdom Yoga Softening here.

BENEFITS Releases and opens the hips, allowing space to breathe and feel. Your hips move significantly during pregnancy due to the pelvis creating space for your baby. Hip openers such as Pigeon Pose create blood flow and energy in the hips, helping to relieve sciatica, hip, and lower back pain.

reflections, clarifications &mementos

week 28

photos or momentos

EXTENDED TABLE TOP WITH PELVIC CIRCLES

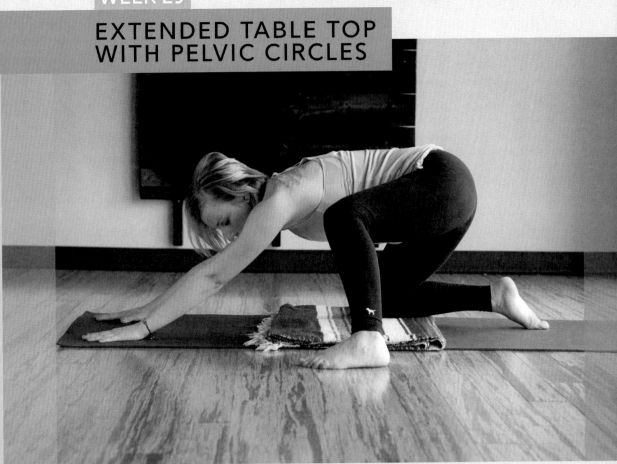

From Hands and Knees, step the left foot out to the side. Soften the left knee, and come into Pelvic Circles slowly, releasing the hips and lower back. Repeat on the right side.

BENEFITS Allows space for a deep release in the hips and lower back. Recommended for all stages of labor and childbirth, including the pushing phase. Opens up the pelvic outlet, creating space for baby.

reflections, clarifications &mementos

week 29

photos or momentos

MODIFIED SIDE PLANK

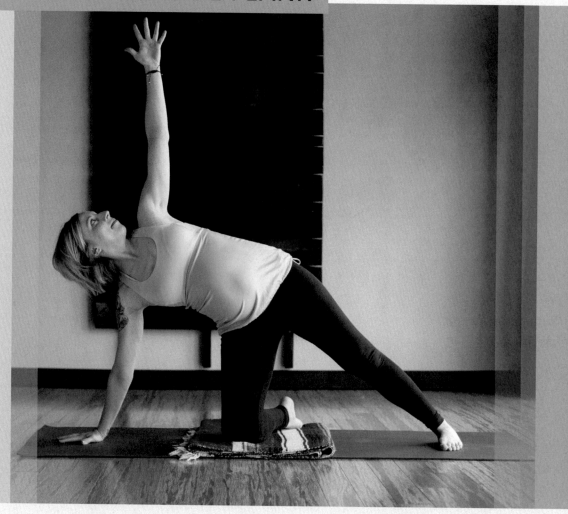

Press your left foot behind you, gently hug your baby up towards your spine, press into your right hand and slide your left foot back in line with your right hip, while pressing your left foot flat on your mat. Inhale the left hand up to the sky. — *three to five breaths* — Release back to Hands and Knees. Take a deep inhale – open up and exhale everything out. Press your right foot behind you, gently hug your baby up towards your spine, press into your left hand and slide your right foot back in line with your left hip, while pressing your right foot flat on your mat. Inhale the right hand up to the sky. — *two to four breaths* — Release back to Hands and Knees. Slowly release into an easy seated position.

BENEFITS Strengthens the arms, shoulders and legs. Gently engages the core.

reflections, clarifications &mementos

week 30

137

photos or momentos

SEATED STRADDLE

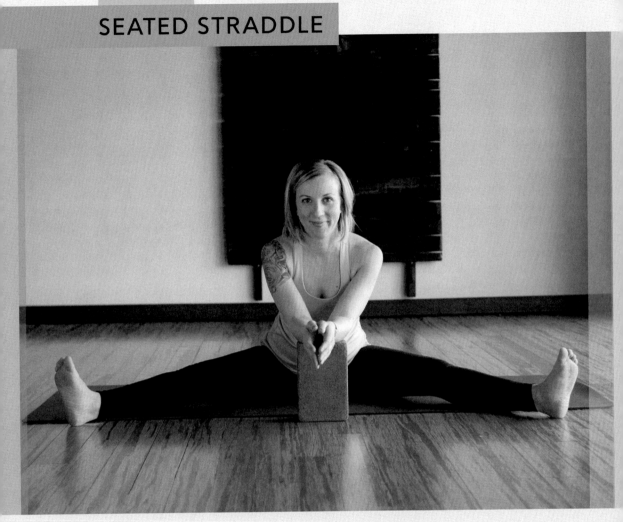

In a seated position, turn and face the side of your mat. Extend your legs open with knees straight and spine tall. Place a block in the center of your legs and inhale your hands to the sky, lengthening your spine. Gently lean forward and rest your forearms or hands on your block. — *five breaths* — This is a great place to practice Birth Wisdom Yoga Softening for labor and childbirth.

BENEFITS Lengthens and strengthens the muscles and ligaments in the pelvic floor, hamstrings and inner thighs.

reflections, clarifications &mementos

week 31

photos or momentos

HEAD-TO-KNEE POSE

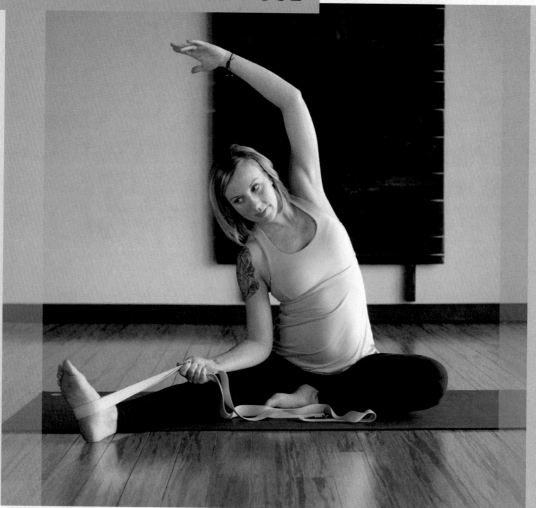

Softly bend your left knee and take the sole of your left foot towards your right inner thigh. Inhale your left hand up to the sky and fold towards your right knee, opening up the left side of your body. — *five breaths* — Repeat on the right side. Practice Birth Wisdom Yoga Softening here.

MODIFICATIONS Use a strap for support and a deeper stretch.

BENEFITS Lengthens and strengthens the muscles in the hamstrings, calves and quadriceps. Releases the shoulders and biceps. Creates an opening in the ribcage and lower back.

reflections, clarifications &mementos

week 32

photos or momentos

SEATED TWIST

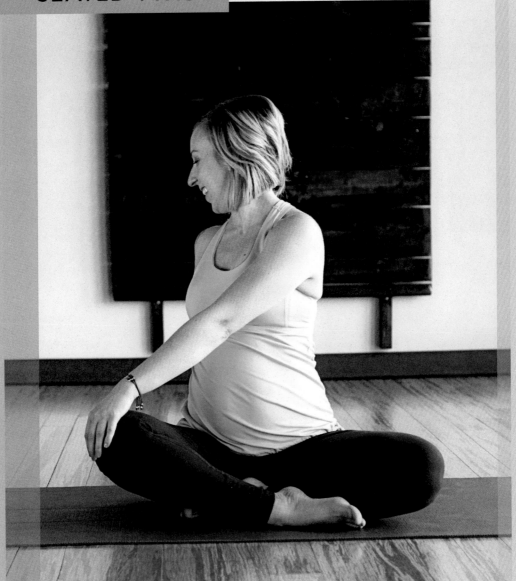

This is a "safe twist" because both of your "sit bones" will stay on your mat. Inhale, lengthen the spine all the way up through the crown of your head — and with your exhale, walk both hands gently to the right side. — *five breaths* — Repeat on the left side.

BENEFITS Encourages optimal digestion while releasing the spine.

reflections, clarifications &mementos

photos or momentos

a collective sisterhood of mothering

> Pregnancy and birth creates a common ground for women from different backgrounds and cultures to come together, sharing our strengths and support.
>
> — *Liz, Birth Wisdom Yoga prenatal and postpartum yoga student*

We have the power as women and mothers to create a supportive, non-judgemental experience for ourselves and the women in our lives. Letting go of perfection and embracing the "messiness of mothering" is a gift we can give to ourselves and our "sisters in mothering." I find that women crave honesty from one another, and it can be very healing and empowering to hear that you are not alone in your daily struggles. By opening up to one another honestly, we can share in a collective power and support system that will feed our souls. Ask yourself today, where you can share your truth about something in your life with a "sisterfriend." We can create our circle of support and power, one honest story at a time.

{affirmations}

I open up and receive the Sisterhood of Mothering.

In gratitude, and in this moment, I am connected to the collective strength of every woman birthing in the world. We breathe, labor and find our own "Divine Feminine" strength together.

I face the pain and work of labor head on, accepting that it is the way to my baby, knowing I have everything I need inside me.

"NATURAL BIRTH" IS WHAT COMES NATURALLY TO YOU

In Birth Wisdom Prenatal Yoga classes, I often say, "Natural birth is what comes naturally to you," meaning that we each have our own unique birth stories and experiences. What each birth will bring to us is a mystery, and the more we can celebrate our paths to our babies, the deeper our connection to trusting our mothering wisdom will be.

I recently had a mom in a Birth Partner Workshop ask me to describe the "best birth" I had attended as a labor and birth doula. I told her that the best birth experiences I have witnessed have been with couples who are informed and empowered to peacefully advocate for what they want in birth. They ask questions, feeling and voicing what they need, and remain fluid to what their birth experience holds for them. Their criterion for judging if they had a "good" or "disappointing" birth experience is not related to whether they opted for pain relief or even needed a C-section. I have found these are the families that feel empowered and exhilarated after labor and childbirth.

It is important to realize that "owning your birth" does not *only* apply to natural births. Statistics from the Center for Disease Control and Prevention show that only 67 percent of women have vaginal births, and fewer than 30 percent of women have natural, vaginal, unmedicated deliveries. We must then ask how we are serving ourselves and each other if we only acknowledge the value of unmedicated, natural birth experiences? When natural birth is our only definition of a "good, empowering birth," we are sadly setting up at least 70 percent of women to feel that they have somehow failed as mothers during their birth experiences.

Being a labor and birth doula and experiencing three natural births myself, I am passionate about the value of a natural birth for mothers and babies. I would certainly love for every mother to have the gift of that experience. Yet after working with hundreds of women in Birth Wisdom Prenatal and Postpartum Yoga classes and as a labor and birth doula, I have found that as a birth community we create sadness for new moms when we do not celebrate and honor each mother's unique path to her baby.

I continue to encourage women to know that "natural birth" is simply what comes naturally to them. I strive to empower women to ask questions, to do research and to know what they want in labor and childbirth. This includes finding out if their care provider is aligned with their vision for the birth of their baby, and further researching their hospital or birthing center's intervention statistics and Cesarean Section rates.

When we can celebrate and honor each woman's birth experience as a sacred path to her baby and mothering, we create space for her to heal and receive the "Pearls of Wisdom" that each birth can bring into her life.

reflections, clarifications &mementos

a collective sisterhood of mothering

What does the "sisterhood of mothering" look like in your life?

_____

_____

_____

What are the experiences of your mother, sisters and/or aunts with childbirth and mothering? How do their experiences relate to you?

_____

_____

_____

_____

Where can you reach out to a "sisterfriend" and share a truth you are experiencing in your life?

_____

_____

_____

What is coming up for you in meditation this week?

_____

_____

_____

Write a letter to your baby.

_____
_____
_____
_____
_____
_____
_____
_____
_____
_____
_____
_____

photos or momentos

SHOULDER SHRUGS

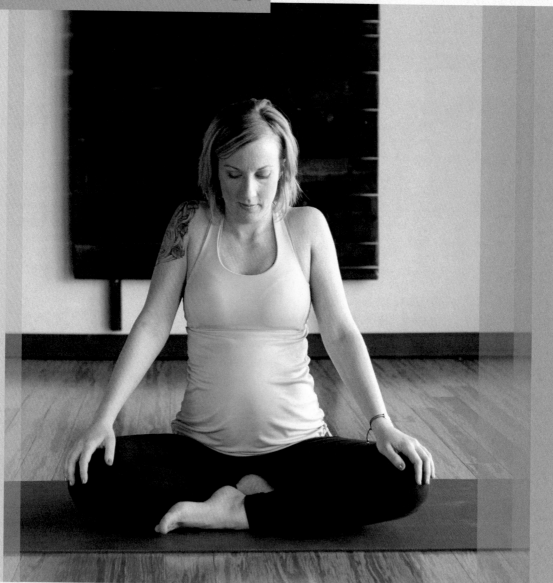

With your breath, take slow circles with your shoulders toward the back of your mat. — *five breaths* — Gently switch to taking the shoulders foward. — *five breaths* —

BENEFITS Allows release of any tension that may remain in the shoulders and upper body.

reflections, clarifications &mementos

week 34

photos or momentos

NECK ROLLS

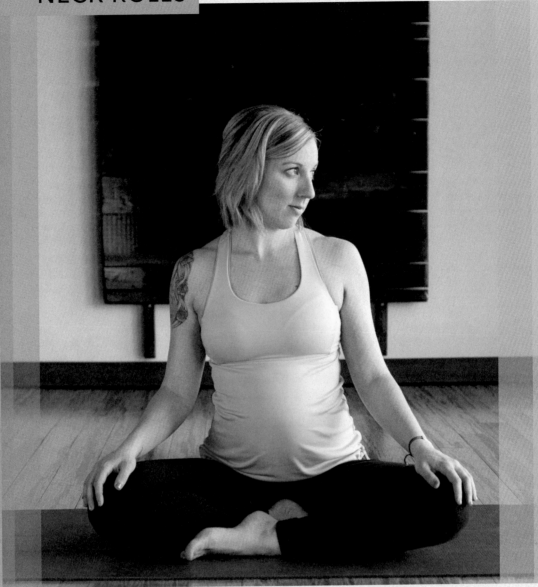

Slowly begin to move your head left and right, gently coming into circles, releasing your neck, taking it slow. — *five breaths* —

BENEFITS Allows release of any tension that may be left in the neck and shoulders.

reflections, clarifications & mementos

week 35

photos or momentos

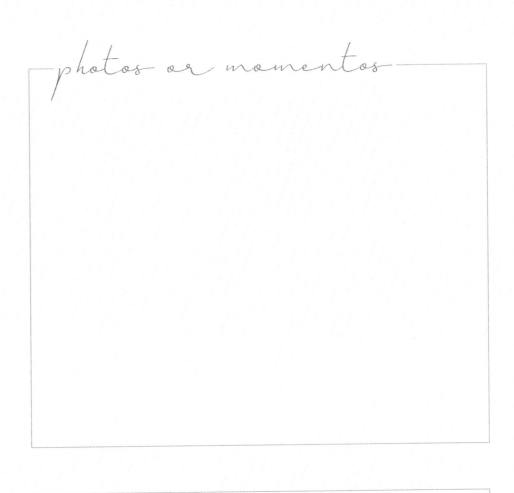

SEATED SIDE STRETCHES

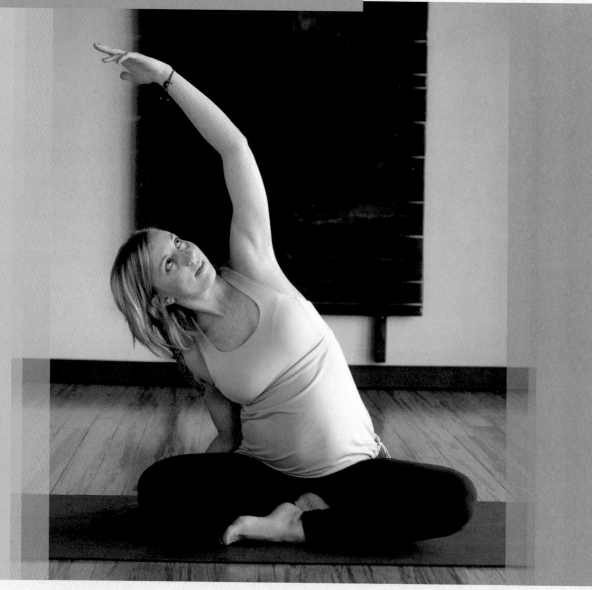

Place your right hand on the floor next to your right hip as you inhale your left hand up to the sky, then take it over to the right. Breathe into the opening in the left side of your body. — *five breaths* — Gently switch sides. Place your left hand on the floor next to your left hip and inhale your right hand up to the sky, then take it over to the left. Breathe into the opening on the right side of your body. — *five breaths* —

BENEFITS Stretches and lengthens the sides of the body, lower back and spine.

reflections, clarifications &mementos

SAVASANA STRETCHES

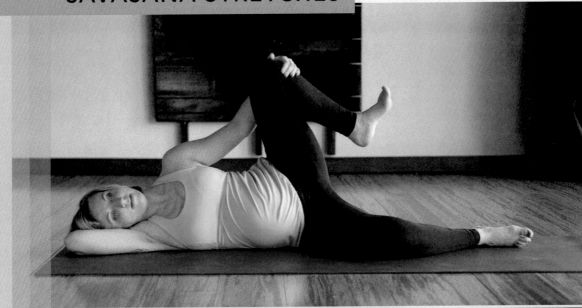

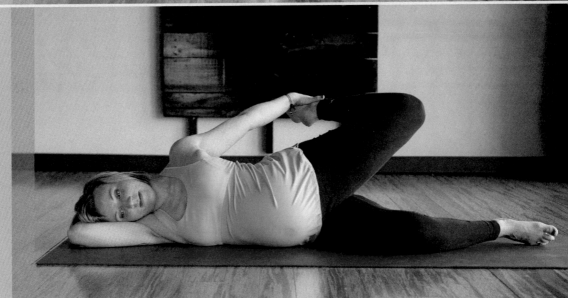

Gently release down to lie on your right side while cradling your head in your right elbow. Soften the left knee and lift it towards your left hip. Drop the left knee down, and take your left heel towards your left glute. Straighten the left leg, and reach for your left big toe or your left hamstring. — *five breaths* — Release to Rocking Happy Baby.

BENEFITS Releases and stretches the hips, quadriceps, hamstrings, calves and lower back.

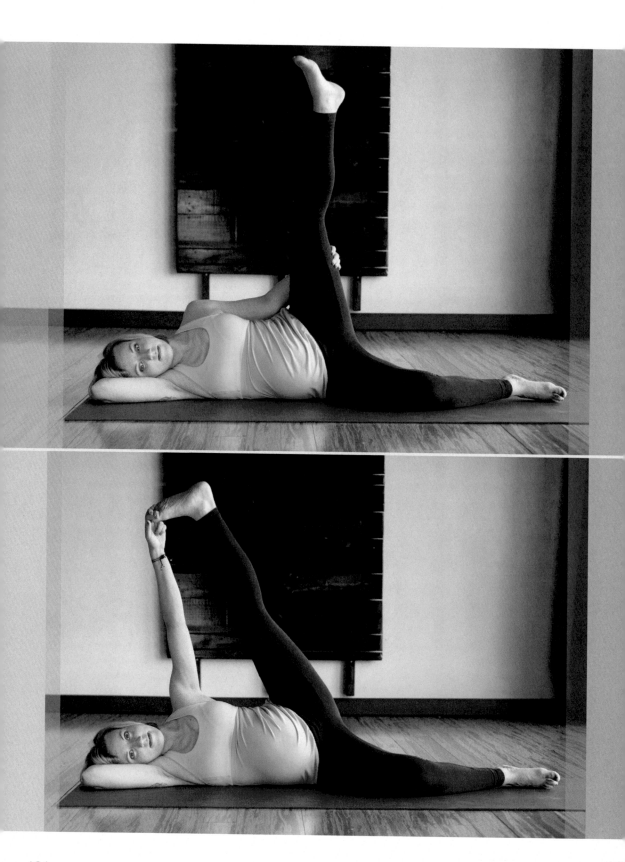

reflections, clarifications &mementos

week 37

photos or momentos

ROCKING HAPPY BABY

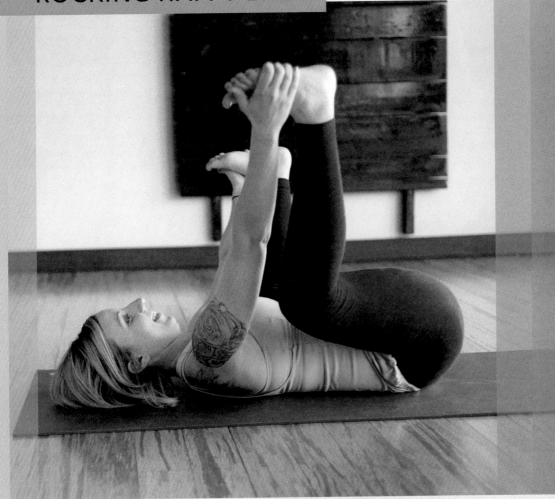

Slowly roll onto your back, with both legs open wide and your knees dropping down towards your hips. Hands come either behind your thighs or on top of your feet. Rock and roll from left to right, giving your spine a gentle massage. When you are ready, rock over to the left side and take your Savasana Stretches there.

BENEFITS Opens the hips and massages the lower back. Provides an easy transition into Savasana Stretches on the left side.

reflections, clarifications &mementos

week 38

photos or momentos

SUPTA BADDHA KONASANA

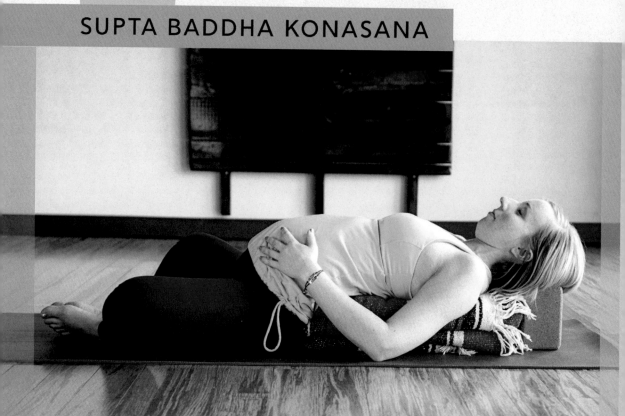

Placing two blankets beginning at your sit bones and extending toward the top of your mat, gently lie down with a block under your head. Soles of your feet are together and knees open wide. If you need more support, place a block or folded blanket under your knees. Place one hand on your baby and one hand on your heart. — *five breaths* —

BENEFITS Creates a gentle, supported stretch in the spine while also allowing blood flow to the hips. Grounding and centering.

reflections, clarifications &mementos

week 39

photos or momentos

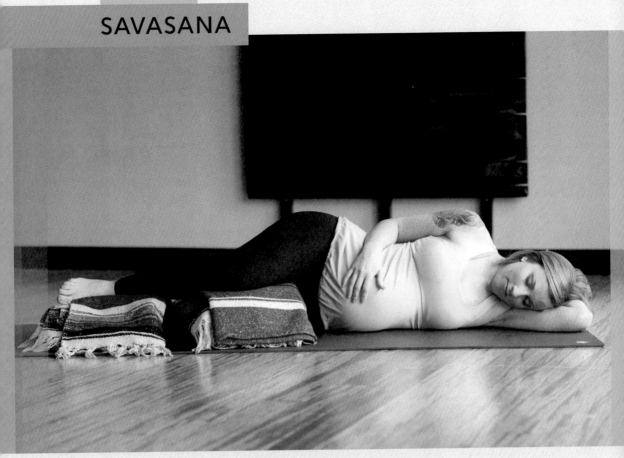

Lying on your left or right side with blankets between your knees and ankles, return to the breath. Soak up this Sacred Space that is just for you and your baby to breathe, feel and connect. — *five breaths* —

BENEFITS Savasana is considered the most important pose in a yoga practice. This is where our body receives the energy of the poses and the breath in our bodies. Our mind and spirit receive what we need here to prepare for labor, childbirth and mothering.

TRANSITIONING TO A SEATED POSITION Take a deep inhale of Love and Gratitude. Allow that feeling to wash over every cell in your body. Take a moment of gratitude that you made it onto your mat today, no matter how busy or tired you are, to do the most powerful thing you can do as a mother for yourself and your family: connecting to your breath. Send your body so much love and gratitude for all the work it is doing to grow and sustain your baby, for your health and strength and for your wisdom and intuition.

Slowly begin to reawaken by gently moving your fingers and toes, eventually meeting in a seated position with hands at heart center.

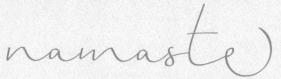

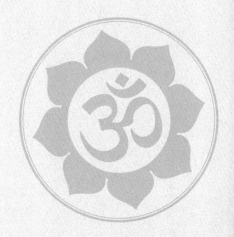

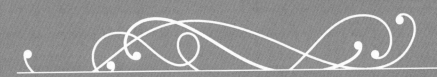

I intend for you to continue using your breath in
your everyday life to connect to and explore each
Birth Wisdom, knowing that your Birth Breathing
and your Birthing Power will be there for you.

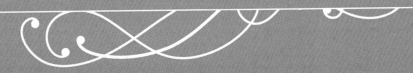

reflections, clarifications &mementos

week 40

photos or momentos

extras

{affirmations}
FOR LABOR AND CHILDBIRTH

In gratitude, I am connected to the
collective strength of every woman
birthing in this moment.
We breathe, labor and find
our own "warrior woman" strength together.

~·~

I have the unlimited power I need to birth my baby.
In harmony with my baby's rhythm,
I let my baby lead the way.

~·~

I see my baby feeling secure, safe and surrounded by
a bright, glowing light of serenity and protection.

~·~

I close my eyes, diving deep into my breath,
where I find the limitless strength and power I need.

I stay focused,
riding each wave of contractions like water.
I am soft. I am fluid.

~·~

After each contraction, I soften my entire body,
completely letting go.

~·~

I only need to make it to the top of each contraction,
knowing that it will release and come back down.
I let each wave go, while saying thank you
for creating a path for my baby.

~·~

I birth with power.

~·~

I see my cervix melting away,
like warm wax dripping down a candle,
making a beautiful passageway for my baby.

BIRTH WISDOM
PRENATAL YOGA FLOW

- Meditation
- Child's Pose
- Legs up the Wall
- Cow Pose
- Cat Pose
- Pelvic Circles
- Bilateral Stretch
- Camel Pose
- Downward Facing Dog
- Mountain Pose
- Child's Pose
- Warrior 1 *right side*
- Prenatal Chaturanga
- Warrior 1 *left side*
- Prenatal Chaturanga
- Warrior 2 *right side*
- Prenatal Chaturanga
- Warrior 2 *left side*
- Triangle Pose to Reverse Warrior *right side*
- Prenatal Chaturanga
- Triangle Pose to Reverse Warrior *left side*
- Prenatal Chaturanga
- Goddess Pose
- Goddess Stretches
- Gate Pose

- Wall Plank
- Slow Dancing *using the wall*
- Half Moon Pose on the Wall
- Tree Pose
- Butterfly / Baddha Konasana
- Bridge Pose
- Pigeon Pose
- Extended Table Top with Pelvic Circles
- Modified Side Plank
- Seated Straddle
- Head to Knee Pose
- Seated Twist
- Shoulder Shrugs
- Neck Rolls
- Seated Side Stretches
- Savasana Stretches
- Rocking Happy Baby
- Supta Baddha Konasana
- Savasana

BIRTH WISDOM PRENATAL YOGA
30-MINUTE FLOW

- Child's Pose
- Hands and Knees
- Cat and Cow
- Pelvic Circles
- Downward Facing Dog
- Mountain Pose
- Warrior 1 *right side*
- Prenatal Chaturanga
- Warrior 1 *left side*
- Prenatal Chaturanga
- Warrior 2 *right side*
- Prenatal Chaturanga
- Warrior 2 *left side*
- Chair Pose *using the wall and a block*
- Wall Plank *using the wall*
- Pelvic Circles *using the wall*
- Tree Pose
- Pigeon Pose
- Extended Pelvic Circles
- Seated Side Stretches
- Seated Twist
- Bridge Pose *with or without a block for support*
- Rocking Happy Baby
- Savasana

labor & delivery

HANDS & KNEES POSE

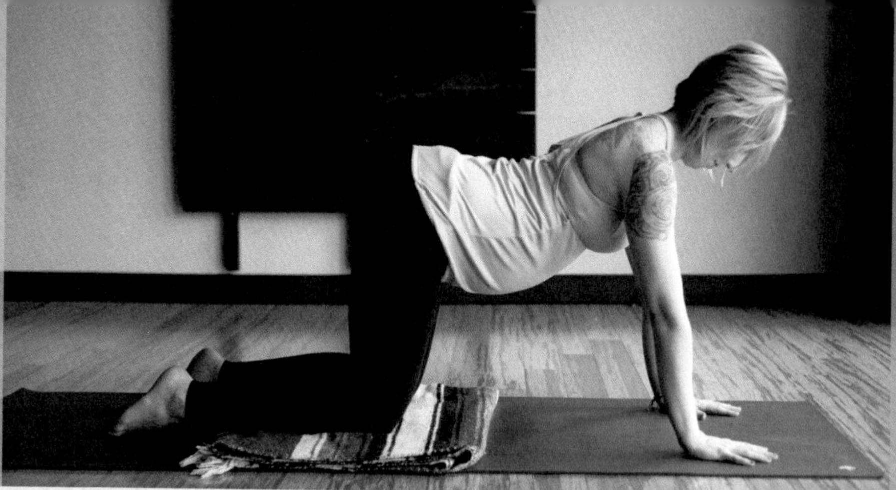

COW POSE

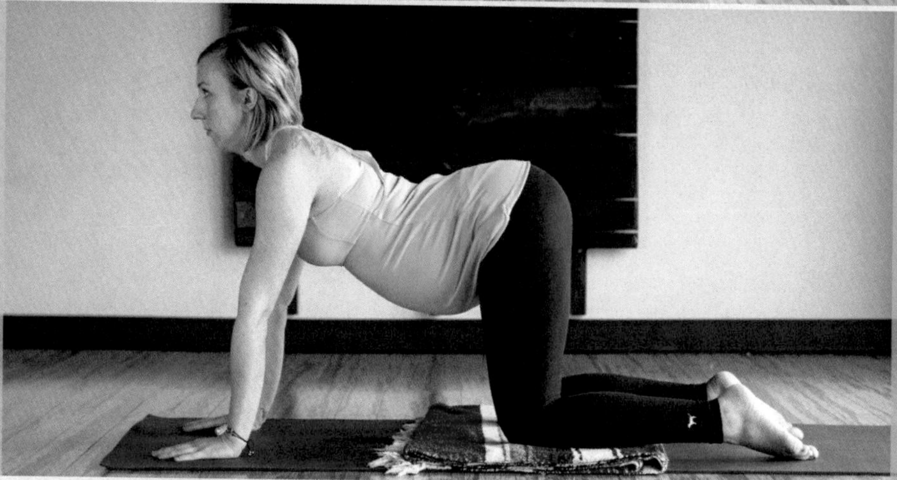

CAT POSE

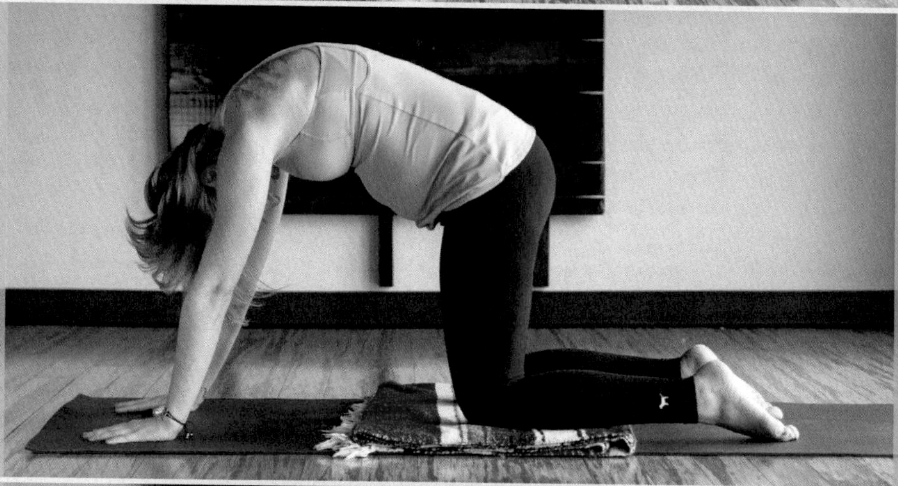

PELVIC CIRCLES

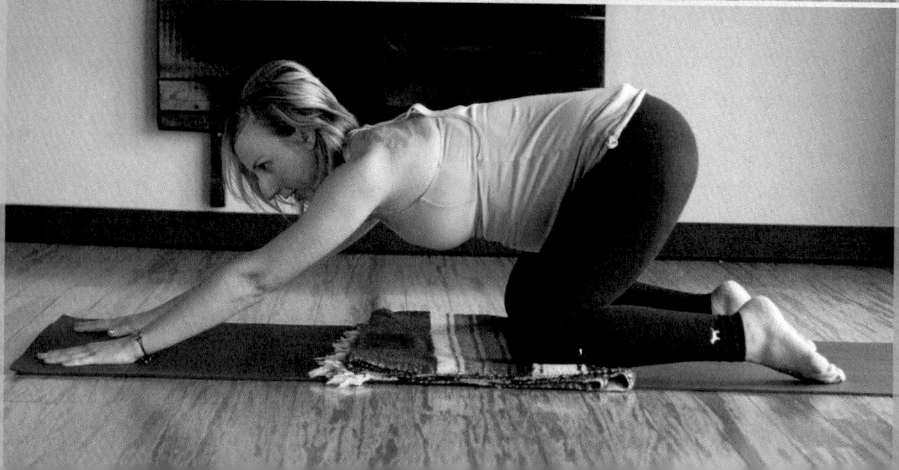

birth wisdom yoga poses to create space for mom and baby in childbirth

HANDS AND KNEES POSITIONS

FOR ALL PHASES OF LABOR AND PUSHING

Practice every day with the Birth Wisdom Yoga Cow / Cat Pose sequence, which includes Pelvic Circles and Extended Pelvic Circles. Not only does this position create more space for baby in the pelvic outlet, but it also helps ensure baby is in an optimal position, *Occiput Anterior,* to fit through your pelvis as easily as possible in labor. In the OA position, baby's head is down and facing toward your back.

Occiput Anterior generally makes movement in the pushing phase easier than the less favored position, "Occiput Posterior," with the back of baby's head facing mom's spine. The Occiput Posterior position can create extreme back pain that can continue in between contractions and sometimes make it difficult for baby to rotate and flow down the birth canal easily. This sequence of poses also allows baby to "float off mom's back" while simultaneously giving the Birth Partner easy opportunity to apply counter-pressure and massage mom's lower back and sacrum.

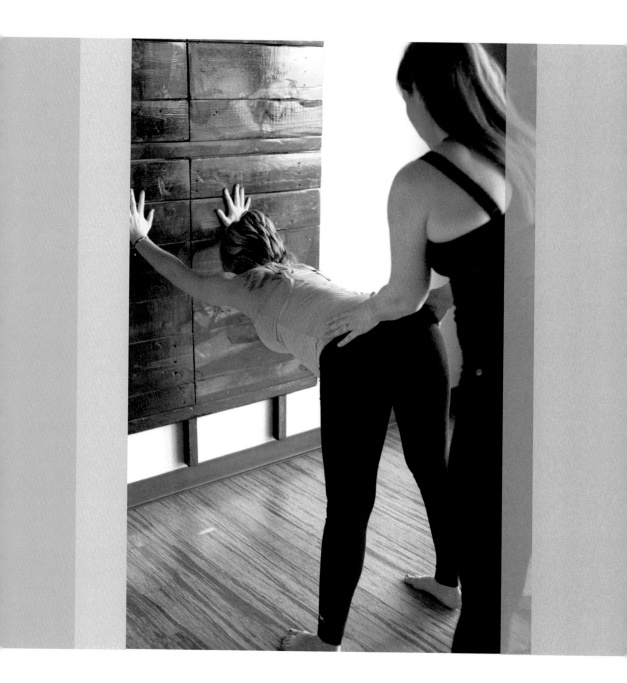

birth partner support & standing positions for labor and childbirth

SLOW DANCING WITH WALKING

This pose is a wonderful way for the Birth Partner to connect with mom through breath and touch, while supporting her physically. Mom has the advantage of gravity working for her and the ability to find pelvic rocking and movement, which can create space for the baby while encouraging him or her to move down the birth canal. Mom can use the wall for support or put her hands around her birth partner's shoulders or neck for support. Slow Dancing With Walking can be alternated with supported squatting in the pushing phase of labor.

Mom can also practice slow dancing in the shower. Her birth partner can apply warm water to her belly or lower back.

LEANING OVER BED

Raise the top of the bed so mom can lean over and put her head on a pillow with her feet wide. This position will create space in the pelvis for baby. Mom can move from left to right and come into pelvic circles, while staying focused on her breath. Leaning Over Bed can be alternated with pushing while in a supported squat.

seated positions for labor

BIRTH BALL

Sitting on the birth ball is essentially a supported squat, which provides optimal space in the pelvic outlet for baby and gives mom a very comfortable place to rest while using gravity to help baby descend. The Birth Partner can sit behind mom, supporting her with the breath, applying counter-pressure and massage. Adjusting the bed so mom can sit on the birth ball and rest her head on a pillow, while alternating with pelvic circles, is often a welcome resting pose that simultaneously supports creating space for baby.

ROCKING CHAIR

This pose provides wonderful counter-pressure on the sacrum while mom relaxes and breathes. It also uses gravity to help baby descend.

TOILET SITTING

Sitting on your toilet can be very comfortable. Once moms are seated on a toilet, they typically don't want to get off! The advantages of sitting on the toilet are similar to the birth ball and rocking chair.

SIDE LYING POSITIONS

Lying on her side can be helpful if mom needs to rest during a long labor. Massaging her hands and feet here can help her to relax.

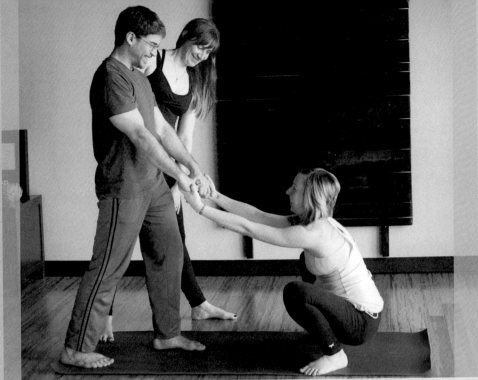

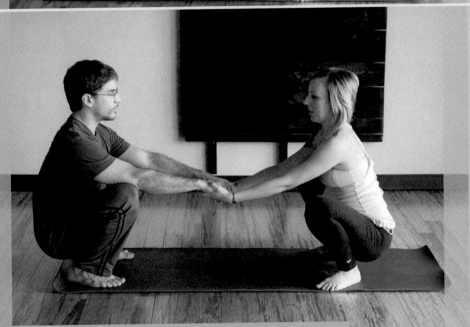

SUPPORTED SQUATTING DURING LABOR

A supported squat can be used during any phase of labor and
pushing, alternated with any movement that feels good to mom.
A squatting bar can also be used for support, while allowing
mom to rest on the bed in between contractions.

labor PAIN

HOW IS IT DIFFERENT THAN AN INJURY?

PURPOSEFUL
You are having a baby.

ANTICIPATED
You anticipate and are prepared.

INTERMITTENT
You get a lot of breaks in between contractions, and you are pain-free most of your labor.

NORMAL
Labor pain is normal.
You are safe, and not in danger.

informed consent questions for your care provider

NAVIGATING PEACEFULLY FOR MOM AND BABY WHEN INTERVENTIONS ARE RECOMMENDED

- **Is this an emergency, or do we have time to talk?**
  If there is time to talk, I recommend that you gather information and then request time alone in the birthing room to decide what feels good for you.

- **What would be the benefit of doing this?**

- **What would be the risk?**

- **If we do this, what other procedures or treatments might we end up needing as a result?**

- **What else could we try first?**

- **What would happen if we waited an hour or two before doing it?**
  This simple question can be the difference between a Cesarean Section or a vaginal birth for mom. Numerous women have shared that this one question was very helpful in avoiding unnecessary medical interventions.

- **What would happen if we didn't do it at all?**

nurturing yourself after your baby is born

1. The first 4-6 weeks require you to sleep when your baby sleeps. If you do this, you will heal twice as fast and feel better physically and emotionally.

2. Soak up the first 4 weeks completely, because you have a newborn for a short amount of time: Babies begin to change and interact more after the first month.

3. Watch your blood flow. You will know if you have "overdone it" by how heavy your flow is. If you are listening to your body and resting when you need it, your flow will be lighter each week.

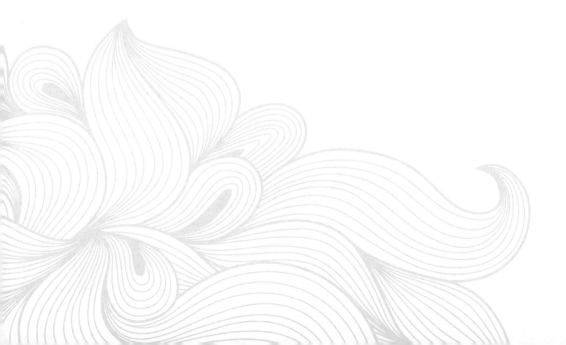

A PHOTO OF
YOU AND YOUR BABY

common ailments &
birth wisdom yoga remedies
quick reference

---

a final message

Dear Birth Wisdom Yoga Sisters,

My hope and dream is that you will gather the Birth Wisdoms here and from your own labor and birth experience and utilize them in your everyday life and mothering. Know that as you walk along your path of womanhood and mothering I am walking and breathing with you.

I am honored to share in and be a part of this Collective Sisterhood of Mothering and Women's Wisdom with you.

Love & Blessings,

Julia

about the author

After earning her Bachelor's Degree in English at the University of California at Davis, Julia Piazza began working as a volunteer labor and birth doula in 2002 at Sutter Davis Birthing Center. After years of supporting women and practicing various forms of yoga, Julia completed her International Doula Certification through Doulas of North America (DONA), a 200-hour Yoga Alliance Certified Yoga Teacher Training and an 85-hour Yoga Alliance Certified Prenatal Teacher Training. Since then, Julia has earned the designation of E-RYT 200 Experienced Registered Yoga Teacher. Her doula work, combined with her love of yoga and appreciation of motherhood, led to the creation of Birth Wisdom Yoga™.

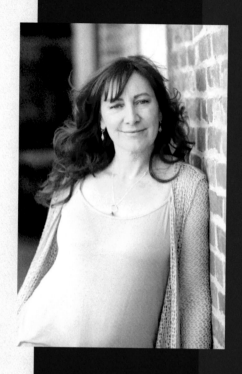

Julia developed the eight Birth Wisdoms over the span of 18 years. While supporting women and their partners through her doula work, Julia noticed universal truths, common "pearls of wisdom" that women discover in labor and childbirth. These epiphanies seemed to connect new mothers with the power and strength needed for mothering and for feeling empowered as a woman.

Julia has worked with hundreds of women and families through various Birth Wisdom Yoga Prenatal and Postpartum Yoga Classes, Birth Partner Workshops, and Prenatal Yoga Teacher Trainings. She currently lives with her husband and three children in Folsom, California, where they enjoy hiking, kayaking, cycling, gardening and ice-skating.

Made in the USA
San Bernardino, CA
16 August 2017